**It's about time the Myths of the Low-Carb Craze were exposed.**

*Why are we being forced to read ridiculous labels that nobody can understand, when the best foods in the world don't have any labels?*

# We've been 'Conned by Carbs'.

**My brilliant H.I. Index is what you need – how much or how badly have humans interfered with your food?**

# the great australian diet

## the atkins alternative

Pulished by
Wilkinson Publishing Pty Ltd
ACN 006 042 173
2 Collins Street
Melbourne Vic 3000
Ph: (03) 9654 5446



First published 2004



National Library of Australia
Cataloguing-in-Publication data:

Tickell, John.

The Great Australian Diet: the Atkins Alternative

ISBN 1 875889 73 6

1. Reducing diets. 2. Health. 3. Exercise. I. Title.

613.25

Page and Cover Design: qgraphics
Printed in Australia by BPA Print Group, Melbourne

Let me ask you these two questions ...

## Question 1

*Do you want your weight loss to be short-term (the quicker the better) or* ***short-term and long-term?***

## Question 2

*Do you want your weight loss to be* ***healthy*** *or* ***unhealthy****?*

*Read on ...*

# Why do we need an alternative?

It is a fact of life that there are not too many people around town who 'go on a diet' and have kept the weight off one year and two years later.

Why?

There are also arguments raging between the disciples of the Atkins-style low-carb, high protein, high fat approach and the many vocal opponents of the diet who say it is really unhealthy and no more effective than any other diet long-term.

There is a war on out there.

Then there are even more arguments about the 'scientific research' behind the diets – cells, ketones, metabolites and other things that scientists talk about.

Diet books also tend to warn people who are pregnant or on medication or have kidney disease or diabetes that maybe the diet is not appropriate for them.

Why?

Is there a problem with what the diet book tells them – is it *dangerous*?

**Nobody** can put up valid arguments against *The Great Australian Diet*, because there is nothing to argue about.

So what's the difference?

> *The Great Australian Diet: The Atkins Alternative* follows Dr John Tickell's ACE skills

> Activity skills
> Coping skills
> Eating skills

It is a 3-pronged attack on life itself.

Equal importance is placed on these three life skills.

Just telling people what or what not to eat does not work.

> *The Great Australian Diet* embraces the EAST versus WEST philosophy

Imagine telling the longest living race of people in the world to eat more fat and protein and to induct a diet with absolutely no fruits or grains!

> *The Great Australian Diet* is based on Dr John Tickell's H.I. Index, not the G.I. Index.

A lot more sensible and much easier to use.

H.I. Index is the level of **H**uman **I**nterference – how much or how badly humans have interfered with your food.

Along the way, you will be astounded by Dr John Tickell's amazing medical breakthroughs and why they make so much sense.

Let's get un-scientific and let's get real!

*The Great Australian Diet* is the best alternative for REAL LIFE.

***The Great Australian Diet: The Atkins Alternative***

# About the author

## DR JOHN TICKELL – A DIFFERENT DOCTOR

Dr John Tickell has an advantage.

You see, his program, *The Great Australian Diet* – 91 DAYS that can CHANGE YOUR LIFE, is a result of real life experiences.

Dr John is a family based Medical Doctor and has spent a lifetime with people.

He knows that women want to be hugged, want to look good, be trim, want their kids to grow up and respect their fellow human beings.

How does he know?

Dr Tickell managed their pregnancies, delivered hundreds of babies and watched their kids grow up.

He has three mature daughters (as well as two sons) all in the health business and he talks to them.

Dr John's wife Sue is a personal trainer who looks after women in their 30s, 40s, 50s and 60s. She knows what women want. Sue knows that women would like to wear a sleeveless dress. **She knows that many women become overweight because of men** – their husbands and partners.

Dr Tickell also understands the Corporate Male.

How come?

Because Dr John is in the Business of Business, planning and building environmentally friendly Living*life* developments.

He knows that men chase success, whatever that is, at the expense of their own well-being and they dismiss the concept of being overweight and not coping – '*I can deal with that later on!*' And Dr John Tickell has been invited by over 2000 companies to speak with their people at meetings and conventions about stress, about life.

Dr John Tickell has another huge advantage.

He travels.

The good Doctor and his two Medical Doctor children have visited in total more than one hundred countries around the world! He knows which races of people live the longest, feel the best, have the lowest rates of cancer, diabetes, arthritis and heart disease. He knows which people are lean, he knows what they eat and how they live their lives.

Dr Tickell is astonished that most health programs emanate from diet 'gurus' who have never been to a country where there are **no** fat people and watched what they eat and what they do from day to day. Cardiologists sit in offices and treat sick people. Scientists sit in laboratories and deal with test tubes and computers.

Dr Tickell would rather seek out and visit and talk with well people, happy people, real people.

That's what *The Great Australian Diet* is all about.

# Table of Contents

# A word from the Good Doctor

My research was very strong and a wonderful help to me as I designed the principles of the exciting *The Great Australian Diet* program.

You see, when something doesn't work LONG-TERM, these are the usual reasons:

### > Too Complicated

Checking indexes, counting grams and ounces, trying to remember all this and getting confused.

### > The Principles Are Wrong

Somebody dreams up a gimmick, everyone jumps on the bandwagon, then the wheels fall off the wagon.

### > Trying Too Hard

Day after day after day.

If it's weight loss you are after, this is what USUALLY happens. You –

- lose fluid quickly
- lose muscle quickly
- lose fat quickly

Then you ...

- regain fluid
- regain fat
- don't put back the muscle

The **RESULT** is you're fatter than when you started. Ultimately it's too hard ... you can't keep going.

**That's why we need *The Great Australian Diet: The Atkins Alternative***

# *The Great Australian Diet* promise

My promise to you … you can be **very successful** at weight loss, both short-term and long-term, if you follow my principles and it is healthy weight loss, NOT unhealthy weight loss.

Once you are living with *The Great Australian Diet*, you will not need the next diet, and the next diet after that, because in 91 Days, you can change your attitude to life.

Attitude is the most important word in the English language. It is so important, I have even reserved space later on to expand on this. Problem is, these days our attitudes are shaped very easily by what goes on around us. For example, we have been pushed into thinking that *exercise* is something that is an add-on to normal life and it is something formal that you have to prepare for, stretch before and then you 'work out', and it is a real hardship. In my program, moving becomes part of your life … it's no big deal (does **walking** sound OK?).

If you want to lose weight, then it MOST CERTAINLY CAN HAPPEN on my program. Again ask yourself these questions:

**Do you want your weight loss to be short-term and long-term? Or short-term (quicker the better) and *not* long-term?**

At least 50 million Americans and two million Australians are on a diet right now. They will all lose weight – some more than others. The fact is however, that the great majority of dieters will put the weight back on, because there is no change in their attitude to life.

My plan works long-term, and if you agree to follow my

principles, you can be lighter, healthier and more energetic, not just 91 Days from now, but one year and many years from now as well.

And what is your answer to the second question?

Do you want your weight loss to be

1. healthy, or

2. unhealthy?

If you answered 2, you are crazy.

Hippocrates, the Father of Medicine, commented some centuries ago that food is our medicine.

How true.

I'm not sure if you are aware of this … food is to the human body both nutritious and healing.

Would you think that bacon, fried eggs and hamburgers are healing us day after day?

The longest living race of people in the world (the Okinawans) eat around five percent (5%) of their food as red meat, poultry, eggs and dairy, whereas these foods make up more than 50% of the American food intake (Australia is not far behind) and the low-carb gurus seem to be pushing us to eat even **more** protein and **more** fat.

I'm going to take you back towards nature (natural). Why do we need to count grams of this and grams of that? We don't. **Why are we being forced to complicate our lives reading labels when the best natural foods (vegetables, fruits, grains and nuts) don't have any labels?**

You may not wish to live until you are 100 (then again, maybe you do, if you look and feel like the sprightly centenarians I have in mind). Make up *your* mind about this as *The Great Australian Diet* program evolves.

I do know what I'm talking about, because I'm a travelling worldly expert at Living*life*, not an office-bound expert or lab technician.

Back to attitudes ...

I repeat, you can be VERY SUCCESSFUL at weight loss, both short- and long-term if you follow my principles; and it is healthy weight loss, NOT unhealthy weight loss. It is as easy as falling off a log if you bring your attitudes and come with me to the *other side* of the world and accept that

- activity is part of life,
- food is to be natural (the way nature intended) and
- there are many ideas we can regularly bring into our lives that can save us from being a 24/7 stress ball.

This is the beginning of you *really* Living*life*.

*Congratulations for being involved.*

Part I

# The Great Australian Diet: The Atkins Alternative

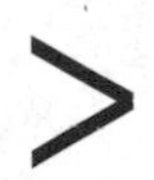

# Why *The Great Australian Diet* works ...

## 91 Days that can Change Your Life

- Because it is Real Life
- Because it is Simple
- Because it is Not Boring
- Because it has been tested on thousands of people with proven results before we let it fly

# My amazing medical breakthrough

This medical breakthrough is the key to your long-term success. *The Great Australian Diet* – 91 DAYS that can CHANGE YOUR LIFE is not 91 Days with the accelerator flat to the floor.

I have realised that the No. 1 reason people fail to change long-term is that they think they can do it and do it and keep on doing it. It doesn't work, so you give up and blow the whole deal.

Listen to me … the limit of human endurance, doing something full on, flat out, nonstop, is around 21 days.

So this is how we are going to tackle *The Great Australian Diet* 91 Day Program.

- **You have a go for 3 weeks**
- **Then you relax and hold for 2 weeks**
- **Then switch back on for another 3 weeks**
- **Then relax and hold for 2 weeks**
- **Then switch back on for another 3 weeks**
- **That's 91 DAYS**

And guess what?

It works!

*'Anyone can lose weight, but why does it come back again?'*

The bottom line is this …

What you really want is **weight loss** which is **long-term** and **weight loss** which is **healthy,** not unhealthy.

Having studied patterns of human behaviour for three decades, I took the strategy associated with success in other fields of human endeavour and applied it to weight loss.

The strategy has been tested over and over again and the proof has arrived – this works, and in my mind it is the only way to lose weight and keep it off – *long-term success.*

The foolproof method is the stepped approach … two steps forward and one step back. In the case of weight loss, the best way the numbers work are three steps forward and two steps back, and even in the 'rest' periods, you don't necessarily go backwards … rather than that, many people just move into a 'holding pattern'.

This is known as my **Switch On, then Hold** approach.

We know that when an athlete achieves a P.B. (that is a personal best, time or distance), there is usually a period that follows when the runner/jumper/swimmer does not keep performing at the same level, but rather consolidates the training and effort that made the P.B. possible.

After this period of consolidation, then we move to the next level of achievement. I'll say it again. The limit of human endurance, doing something full-on, is around 21 days.

That's the reason most dieters fail. Like I said before – they think they can just keep on doing it. They can't, so they give up and go back to their old ways. The pack of cards collapses big time.

So the weight comes off, the weight goes back on – off, on – off, on.

Doesn't work.

The medical breakthrough is all about the **Switch On, then Hold** approach – the sensible way to Personal Best.

This does work.

At the risk of repeating myself, *The Great Australian Diet: The Atkins Alternative* is successful, because it locks into a natural pattern of human behaviour.

> **You have a go for 3 weeks**
> **Then you relax and hold for 2 weeks**
> **Then switch back on for another 3 weeks**
> **Then relax and hold for 2 weeks**
> **Then switch back on for another 3 weeks**
> **That's 91 DAYS.**

Remember Kenny Rogers and *The Gambler*?

*'You've got to know when to hold 'em,*
*Know when to fold 'em,*
*Know when to walk away,*
*Know when to run ...'*

So, this is how *The Great Australian Diet* works – 91 Days that can Change Your Life.

And by the way, during the **Hold** periods of the 91 Day program, if you happen to put back on 50% of the weight you've lost in the previous 3 weeks, then that immediately triggers the next 3 week **Switch On** period.

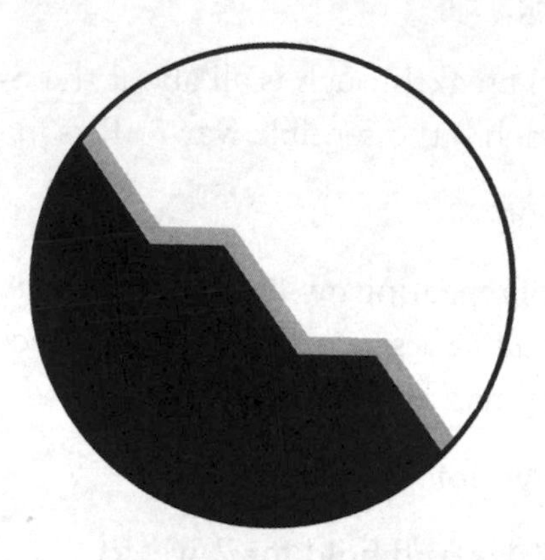

It means you haven't been 'holding' too well. It's a learning process. It takes 21 days to break half a bad habit or conversely, form half a good habit.

# Dramatic differences

I've already explained the simple yet amazing breakthrough I call **Switch On, then Hold ...**

Add to this the most sensible approach of all time – the way you choose the food you eat.

## > BASIC Foods and BONUS Foods

There are two food groups in the world – not four, not five food groups, but two.

BASIC Food is Plant Food – vegetables, fruits, grains, nuts and seeds.

BONUS Food is everything else!

## > TWO-THIRDS, ONE-THIRD

You will be eating at least 2/3 BASIC Food, less than 1/3 BONUS Food and very little refined food.

## > The AMAZING RULE of 15

We are aiming to eat small portions of 15 different Plant Foods each day. Not the whole thing, just little nibbles here and there. Variety is the name of the game ... and it's easy!

## > My REVOLUTIONARY H.I. INDEX

Everyone has heard of the G.I. Index. Well, the H.I. Index is a far safer and more intelligent approach.

The H.I. Index will **revolutionise** the way we choose the food we eat. H.I. is the Human Interference Index and is a measure of how much or how badly humans have interfered with our food.

*The Great Australian Diet* has so many successful breakthroughs that provide you with the knowledge and the tools to achieve success.

It is **new** and it is all good.

If you follow the program, you **can** succeed and achieve **healthy, long-term weight loss**.

# East versus West

I recently travelled to Okinawa to again check on the longest living race of people in the world.

The Okinawan Islands sit off the southern end of Japan, and the percentage of centenarians or hundred-year-olds is the highest of anywhere on this planet.

I can hear some people mumbling that they don't want to live to 100 because their perception of a 100-year-old is that of a withered person sitting motionless in a chair in a rest home.

Well I have news for you. The Okinawan Elders are sprightly people who look more like they are in their 70s and they are sound in body and mind.

This trip to Okinawa however, made me very sad.

One of the photographs I took said it all ... a picture tells a thousand words.

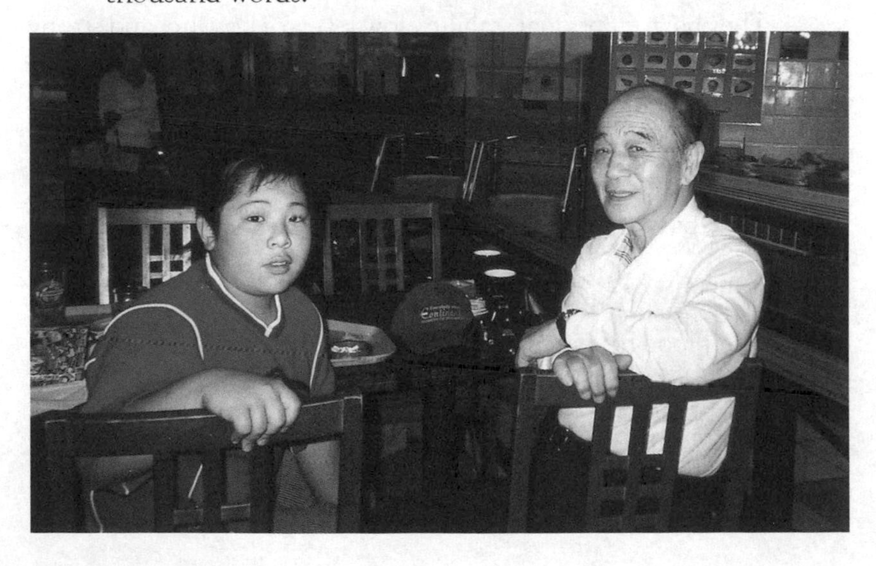

There was the elderly gentleman, lean and healthy, sitting with his grandchild who was not lean at all.

The little kid was fat – apologies – obese (more politically correct).

None of the Okinawan Elders are overweight, and I mean none, nil, zero.

They don't eat Western food with a poor H.I. Index, but their youngsters do. I'll give you more detail on the H.I. Index later.

The incidence in the older folk of heart troubles, diabetes and hormone-dependent cancers like breast cancer, prostate cancer and bowel cancer is extremely low, and there are no rest homes because they don't need them.

What else do they do?

They move and work physically every day.

They catch and eat fish most days – they eat a **huge variety** of vegetables, grains and fruits.

They have emotional stability, low levels of hostility and strong social integration within a village system (they don't hate their neighbours).

They don't 'retire'.

They have a saying ... '*nuchi gusui*'

It means '*May your food (and lifestyle) heal*'.

Their food heals because of the amazing abundance of micro-nutrients available to their human machines.

And yet the Western Way is chock-a-block full of 'Human Interfered with' foods which are virtually devoid of nutrients but still full of calories.

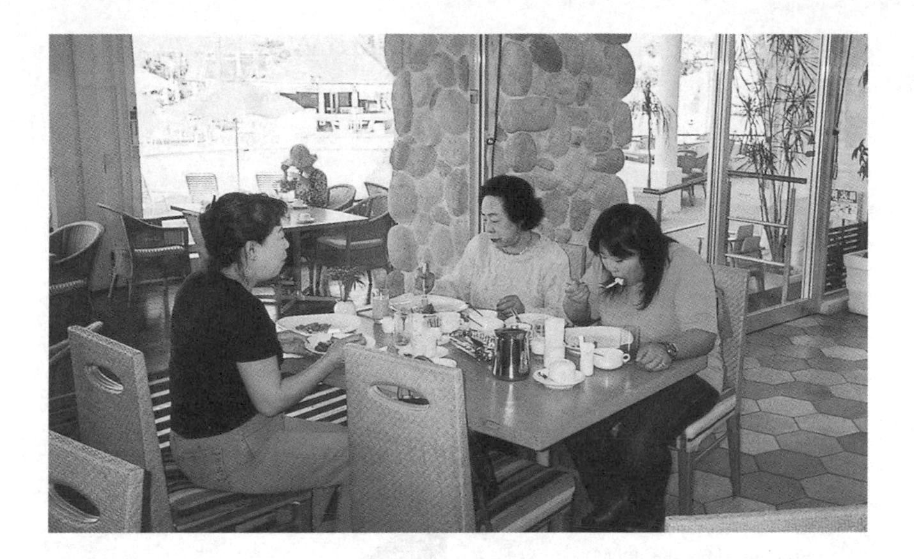

Check out the above photo of three generations of women.

Note the shift in body weight and also note the utensils – chopsticks for grandmother and for grandchild, a fork (shovel) in right hand.

The proof is in the pudding (so to speak). Need I say more?

Why do I propose an alternative to the Western Way?

One reason is that the anti-carb gurus are 'inducting' our diet with more fat and protein, more red meat, poultry, cream, butter and absolutely no fruit or grains.

Imagine telling the longest living race of people in the world to eat like that!!

My research shows me that a comparison of the eating habits of Okinawan Elders and the Western Way in the US goes something like this:

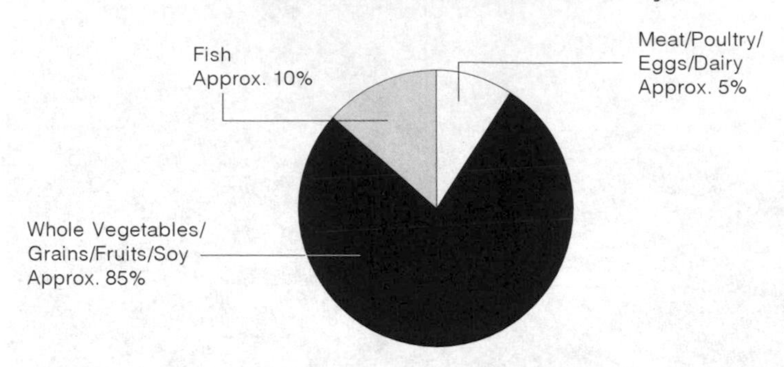


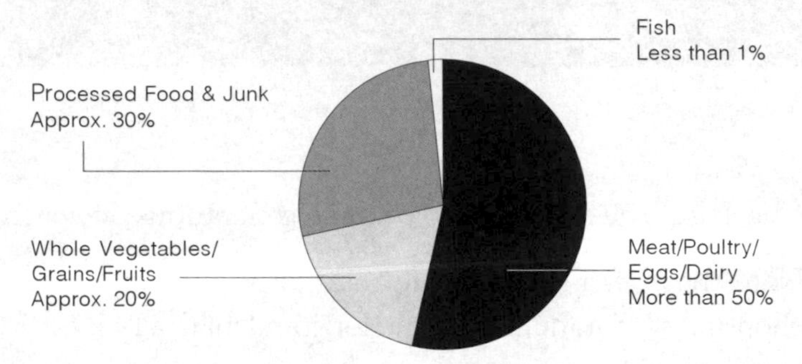


PLEASE show me all the sprightly, lean 80, 90 and 100-year-olds with lots of energy and *very* low rates of diabetes, heart attacks and cancer that eat the Western Way.

*The Great Australian Diet* sways the pendulum towards the Eastern Way ... at least two-thirds of the way to the Eastern Way.

You can eat anything you like, but at least 2/3 BASIC Food and maximum 1/3 BONUS Food – Rule No. 1.

Are you with me?

GOOD.

# Myths of the low-carb craze

- The Western World has been 'Conned by Carbs' – low carbs, no carbs, impact carbs, non-impact carbs, net carbs. Carbs, schmarbs ... listen up folks ...
- Why do we need to invent low-carb mania when our maker has already produced the perfect nutritional smorgasbord?
- The longest living races of people in the world eat mainly carbohydrates (low H.I.), some protein and little fat. They are lean and energetic. So why would you want to do the exact opposite?
- By the way, carbs are not carbs, they are carbohydrates – $CH_2O$ If you leave out the hydrate bit, you are missing the $H_2O$ (the water), which is ***very*** important.
- The manufacture of 'low-carb' products is motivated by you-know-what. But most of them FAIL the basic H.I. test – the Human Interference test.
- Carbohydrates are great fuel for the human body and are clean burning – they end up as **glucose, water** and carbon dioxide, which you breathe out. You breathe in oxygen ($O_2$) and breathe out carbon dioxide ($CO_2$).
- Glucose feeds the brain, the nerve systems and your muscles. Fat doesn't feed them, glucose does. Glucose comes from carbohydrates. If you want energy and if you want to think smart, you need carbohydrates.
- Real carbohydrates (Plant Foods) contain many, many more vitamins and minerals than fat and protein. These nutrients pump up the immune system and a strong immune system

dramatically reduces your risk of colds, influenza and cancers – in fact, all diseases.

> Nobody associates the ingestion of real carbohydrates (low H.I. – vegetables, grains, fruits) with human disease, whereas high blood pressure, heart disease, stroke, cancer, diabetes, arthritis and osteoporosis **are** associated with high intake of fats and protein.

Ever heard anyone say this?

'*My husband died of a heart attack because he ate too many beans*' ...

'*She got cancer because she ate too much pineapple*' ...

> Scientists tell me that the more fat and protein you eat, the more calcium is leaving your body – not good.

> The people in the world who eat low fat, low protein, high real carbohydrates, have the **lowest** rates of cancer.

High fat, high protein communities have the **highest** rates of cancer ... your choice.

> The idea that the Glycaemic Index (G.I.) of one particular food is the dominating factor in deciding whether it should or should not be eaten is ridiculous.

You could be excused for thinking there is a guy at the gateway to the stomach and intestines calling out the numbers and directing traffic.

'*Pineapple – 94 – straight into the blood stream*' ...

'*Soybeans – 25 – hang around here for a while*' ...

The G.I. makes you freak out just because you see a number higher than 45 or 55 or whatever. The G.I. of one thing or another is irrelevant if you are eating foods that have low human interference.

- All carbohydrates are sugars – they are sugar molecules stuck together. There are three basic sugars – glucose, galactose and fructose. For example, sucrose or table sugar is glucose and fructose stuck together. When humans interfere with natural or real carbohydrates, they 'refine' and 'process' foods so that they go into the blood steam real fast and cause huge demands on insulin production. (The Diabetes Chapter says it all.)

- If you concentrate mainly on real foods (not messed up by humans) then you don't need to worry about G.I. numbers. Here are a few fantastic tips to slow down the impact of your food being absorbed too quickly. And if you are losing sleep over watermelon or pineapple because of a high G.I. number, simply add a low G.I. number food and eat them together – hey presto – it all slows down, e.g. add low fat yoghurt or skim milk – both in the low 30s. But why get stressed about it?

Slower food absorption is good, so to achieve this, you can

- add a little olive oil
- add some lemon or vinegar
- add some low fat yoghurt or low fat sour cream
- add lentils, chickpeas, soybeans
- add some low fat grated cheese
- add more FIBRE to your meal

When humans interfere with food and refine it and process it, they take out the fibre and stuff up the food, e.g. white bread. Then they put on the label 'vitamin enriched' or 'vitamin fortified'. Why did they take the vitamins out in the first place? But so called white bread is NOT bread. Bread is whole grains. Make sure your rice is whole grain rice, like it is in Asia.

> FIBRE is also carbohydrate. It slows down the absorption of your food – a lot of fibre is indigestible so it helps to sweep much of the muck and toxins and cholesterol out of your intestines as it passes through. Fibre acts like a sponge. You may wish to use a **little** of the Indian grain called psyllium to help you along – it is very high in fibre, but take it easy.

P.S. Vegetables, grains and fruits have heaps of fibre – fat has zilch.

> Once the glucose is in your blood, it is used as fuel for your brain and muscles, and the energy provided by this sugar can actually be stored in your muscles and liver.

Now there's a good idea.

If your 600 or so muscles were used now and then, they would be bigger, more efficient, and you would soak up a lot more glucose from your blood. Fat cannot soak up glucose like muscles can – not even in the same ballpark. So toned, strong muscles and less fatty tissue in your body mean more energy and less chance of diabetes.

Walk, walk, walk and do your SBWs (strengthening exercises).

> For a bit of a smile, have a Captain Cook (look) at these G.I. Ratings:

| G.I. RATINGS | ATKINS | SOUTH BEACH |
|---|---|---|
| Brown Rice | 55 | 79 |
| Banana | 52 | 89 |
| Watermelon | 72 | 103 |
| Baked potato | 85 | 158 |
| Sweet potato | 54 | 63 |
| Chick peas | 33 | 47 |
| White bread | 70 | 101 |

Confused? ... I am.

Who do you believe? Who cares?

H.I. not G.I. – *The Great Australian Diet.*

Are you tired of carbs yet? Just hang in there. I have one more thing for you.

Carbohydrates are sugars stuck together and sugars are carbohydrates but they don't call them carbs unless more than two sugars are stuck together, then you're allowed to call them carbs. What a laugh!

Whoever invented the label (not libel) laws should be made to explain them to a bunch of people like me because they don't make sense. It's just crazy. If fruit had a label (thank goodness it doesn't) it would say 'lots of sugar in here' – because fructose (fruit sugar) is not a carbohydrate because only one sugar is stuck to itself. So the low carb guys get hysterical and say you can't eat fruit in the first few days or weeks because it has sugar in it, but fructose has a G.I. of only 23! Can't eat fruit, huh?

I want to be healthy, so I eat fruit.

I challenge any author of a low-carb, high fat diet to go to the other side of the world, not once, but dozens of times, watch the long-living, lean people, then call me and tell me what they eat is wrong.

I won't wait by the 'phone.

# What went wrong with the Western Way?

> ACTIVITY

- We don't move

> COPING

- Life is too complex

> EATING

- Human interference – we take good food and wreck it
- Oversized servings makes for oversized people
- Lack of variety = boring

We forget the BASIC Food and replace it with BONUS Food.

# The Land Down Under – which way to go?

Australia is a lucky country … beautiful beaches, clean cities, stunning rainforests, stark deserts, the wonders of the reef.

We are fun-loving people for sure, but we are now at the crossroads and need to ask ourselves the big questions:

> *Do we join the rest of the Western World, gradually breaking down our personal systems, or do we go back to basics and learn how to really live again?*

> *Do we continue to listen to the quick-fix merchants? If their miracles work so well, why is there another and another?*

> *Do we stick bandages all over a broken down system or do we go back a way and get the basics in place?*

One thing is for sure.

The answer to weight loss and health does not lie within the US, Australia, or any other Westernised culture.

The researchers are doing more and more 'studies' on which food does what to whom and the relationship between in-grown toenails and low sex drive, and while this goes on, we get fatter and unhealthier.

As well, you have these bizarre concepts that tell us that what we eat is supposed to depend on our star sign or our blood type! People actually believe that stuff. C'mon, get real!

Now they are 'inventing' ways to take fat and sugar out of foods and stick other goodies into other foods. For goodness sake, leave food alone!

Then they tell us not to eat carbs ... how crazy is that?

The best two foods in the world, vegetables and fruits, **are** carbohydrates.

So is there an answer?

The answer my friend is blowin' in the wind and the wind has lifted me and carried me to all corners of the globe.

For Australians right now, the scales are firmly tilting to the West.

But we are so lucky to be geographically where we are.

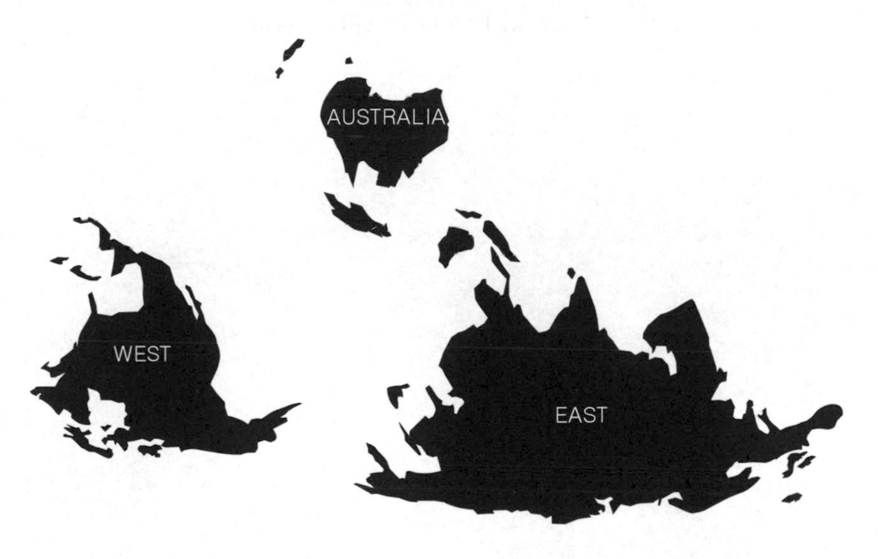


PS. Because Australia is not Europe (we are the Land Down Under), EAST is WEST and WEST is EAST for us. Don't worry about it ... just read on.

We can choose to swing towards the West or the East.

I say we go EAST.

It's more interesting, more fun and far, far healthier.

There lies the answer.

I have not based my research on a nation of overweight people and watched what they do wrong – I have based my research on nations of long-living, normal-weighted people with low rates of cancer, heart disease, diabetes and arthritis and watched what they do right.

This is my choice and I trust it will be yours.

# Why 91 Days?

Because 10 days doesn't work and you know it.

And 14 days and 28 days don't work either.

Let me ask you this.

Are you prepared to do something decent for yourself, for your body and your mind, over the next few weeks ... or are you going to wimp it and walk away from this golden opportunity and wait for the next 10-day miracle cure?

There are no miracles in the business of self-improvement – and that's the truth.

Is it really worth the effort you say?

Well 91 Days is such a short period of time compared to the rest of your life.

Is it a matter of life or death?

Yes it is – but what's equally important is the **quality** of the rest of your life.

# Attitude

Without doubt, **attitude** is the most important word in the English language.

And the sad fact of life is that more and more people today look at the downside rather than the upside.

The weather forecast is 'partly cloudy' rather than 'partly sunny'.

We wake to a new day and instead of celebrating the fact we are alive and can do good things today, we worry about what is going to go wrong.

We don't want our kids to play ball in the street or ride their bicycles to school these days because we are scared of the bad things that may happen, so we wrap them in cotton wool and they suffer.

Can we blame someone apart from ourselves?

Top of the list would have to be the media.

People listen to or watch 'The News' on the hour – every hour.

There is no good news (except for sport) … murders, rapes, crashes, fires, viruses, cowards bashing and stealing from elderly people, corporate fraud. Why would anyone in their right mind need regular doses of that?

George Burns was a hero of mine.

He had a great attitude to life. A positive thought for every occasion.

He was even upbeat about being in his 90s … *'You're not bothered by insurance salesmen any more'*.

What we need is a change of attitude, and the way to do it needs to be simple because you don't want to be confused while you are changing your attitude.

# We don't control our lives – our lives control us

Here is a list of just some of the people/things that control us in varying degrees.

> Television

> Advertising

> Multi-National Companies

> Kids

> Clocks

> Fashion

> Enemies

> Fear

> Banks

> Stock Markets

> Retirement Experts

> Routine

> Your Taste Buds

Are you pleased about this or not?

Maybe we need a little time out to reflect on who or what is controlling our lives.

# About women

Please don't get upset with me for writing this – all the information came from women.

> My wife Sue tells me that women are concerned about their thighs and their bottoms, about their stomachs and about their arms, especially the flabby bit that wobbles at the back of the arms. If this body part is tight, wearing a sleeveless dress is OK.

> Women don't like to leave any food on the plate if it has been served for them at a private home because that's insulting to the person who cooked or prepared it.

> Women can easily talk to other women about stuff like relationships and diets. Men can't do that.

> Young women now begin having menstrual cycles around five or six years earlier than they did a few decades ago. Why?

More fat, more hormones, more fast food and less activity. This is a pity because the experts are thinking that the earlier start of menstrual cycles is one of the reasons for a higher risk of breast cancer in the Western World.

(Interesting that menstruation, menarche and menopause all start with 'men'!)

> If a woman gives you food and you don't eat it, there must be something wrong.

*'You must eat it all, clean your plate – think of the starving children.'*

My response – *'Send it to them – I've had enough, thank you'.*

- Women dress to impress other women – 'looks good, very classy'.
- If a woman dresses to attract a man, the neckline goes down and the skirt goes up, but then other women think that's not nice.
- Women want to be thinner than men want them to be.
- Women work a lot more away from home than they used to because women now have careers.

  I don't have a problem with this, but the researchers tell me that working women don't prepare as much food at home or work around the house as much or run after children as much and they are therefore burning a hell of a lot less calories.
- '*Never trust a skinny chef*' is on a plate that hangs in our kitchen.
- Women used to do all the cooking except in restaurants. A 'good cook' in the past was totally different to what a 'good cook' is now.
- Women usually are concerned with their man putting on weight and are worried about him having a heart attack because men have a lot of heart attacks.
- Women say things like '*You need to do something about yourself*'.

  Well, get them involved in *The Great Australian Diet: The Atkins Alternative,* over the next 91 DAYS.
- The fantastic thing about *The Great Australian Diet* is this – we know it works for women as this has been proven over and over again – but now we also know it works for men as well. The male members of **Rex Hunt's Fat Club** have lost substantial amounts of weight without going hungry.

## About men

- Men couldn't really care less about putting on weight and they aren't worried about having a heart attack except for a couple of days after their best mate drops dead.
- Men have several mates, so if one mate moves on, there are others to have a drink with.
- It is embarrassing not to complete a 'shout' or a round of beers and you can't leave till that's happened.
- Men talk to other men about sport, money and sex. That's not a revelation.
- Men who are getting fat have higher blood pressure but they don't know until something goes wrong because there are no symptoms of high blood pressure, and men don't go to have their blood pressure (or their prostate) checked.
- Men struggle with life balance – they have problems managing the amount of time spent juggling work, family and personal well-being. Men watch their kids play sports and they hope like hell the kid is better than they were.
- Men go through 'menopause' but instead of getting hot flushes they worry about success and the meaning of life and where it's all heading, and can they 'perform'.
- Married men live longer than single men, but single women live longer than married women.

The life chapter of a man is somewhat shorter than the life chapter of a woman. It doesn't need to be.

# The greatest machine on earth – the human machine

So how is your great machine today?

Is the pump in fine working order?

Are the pipes in good shape?

Is the brain box sparking and firing on all cylinders?

Are the 600 muscles and 180 joints well tuned?

Are you having some fun?

Are you really alive?

Or is the machine gradually sludging up, rusting, creaking, groaning and on its way to grinding to a halt?

And are the excess pounds of fat dragging you down so you're tired and losing energy?

You can reverse the trend in just **91 Days** with *The Great Australian Diet*.

Great!

# Is *The Great Australian Diet* difficult?

No, it's not difficult – it's fun.

> Would you like to look younger and trimmer?

> Would you like less stress, more energy and enthusiasm for life?

> Would you like to feel better with less aches and pains?

> Would you like to sleep better and be more in control?

> Would you like to laugh at life a little more?

Then the bottom line is this …

You eat, you drink, you rest, you walk, you stretch, you lift a few things and you get back in touch with life.

It really isn't a huge hassle.

So, let's do it.

Part II

# The ACE skills - A sneak preview

>

# ACE

I'll give you a sneak preview of *The Great Australian Diet* program – 91 DAYS that can CHANGE YOUR LIFE.

The basis for the success of *The Great Australian Diet* is that it hits on the total spectrum of life.

**Alternative**

You pick up the usual 500 page diet book and 498 pages tell you what to eat, there is one page on exercise and one page on how to run your life. One famous diet program even says that exercise is not necessary! That gave me a really good laugh. What a load of hogwash.

**Reality**

*The Great Australian Diet* is based on the three core skills of self-management –

> Activity skills

> Coping skills

> Eating skills

The **A C E** skills.

The reason the ACE program is so successful? ... Equal weighting is placed on these three important aspects of life.

# Activity skills

## Guidelines

> **1%**

1% – you MUST move for a minimum dose of one percent of your life – Burning Rubber

> **SBW**

Strong is Better than Weak – Strengthening Exercises

> **OUMs**

Other Useful Movements – Stretching Exercises

# Coping skills

> Pressure is on the outside.

Stress is on the inside.

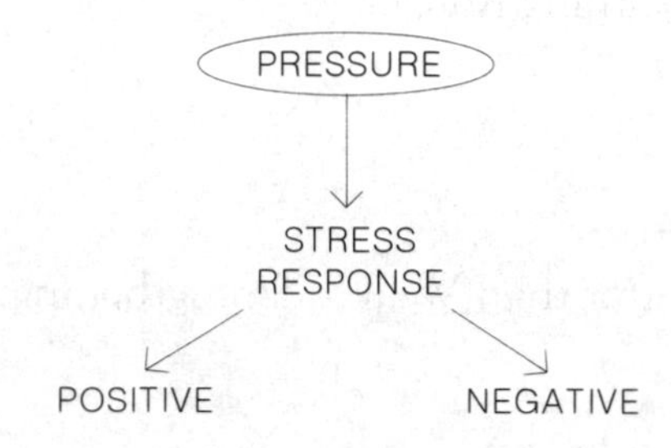


> Escape from the

Pressure Cooker of Life

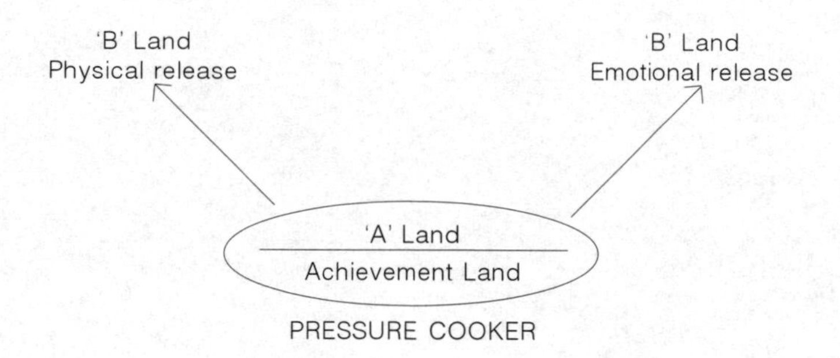


> Hakuna Matata – it means '*no worries*'.

# Eating skills

## Guidelines

> **Basic** **Bonus**

There are two food groups in the world

BASIC FOODS (Plant) and BONUS FOODS (Non-Plant)

> **2/3** **1/3**

2/3 – 1/3 Two-thirds Plant Food, and One-third other stuff

> **R.O.15**

The Rule of 15 – nibbles of 15 different Plant Foods each day

> **H.I. Index**

H.I. Index, not G.I. Index - The level of human interference

# Part III

# Activity, Coping & Eating uncensored

>

Activity >

Coping

Eating

# Activity

> We don't walk enough

> We don't lift enough

> We don't move enough

Our human machines have approximately 600 muscles and 180 joints and we hardly use any of them.

What happens to a piece of machinery when we don't use it for long periods of time? That's right, it ceases to function properly. Our body, the greatest machine ever invented, is no different.

Inactivity creeps up on you – the systems are shutting down – then something goes wrong. Bang! Who is to blame?

The Activity part of *The Great Australian Diet: The Atkins Alternative* is crucial.

It's not difficult. Climbing Mount Everest is not part of the deal. Moving regularly **is** part of the deal.

Keep at it and it gets easier. And you feel better ... and better.

# One step at a time

A cliché for sure, but how true!

Walking is great, especially if you're carrying an extra brick or two around the tummy or thighs, and walking means less strain on the joints as well.

If you're in good shape, you may want to walk and jog, but don't push too hard.

You might walk a lot as part of your work, but then again you probably don't.

Most of us travel to work on wheels – not bicycle wheels, but on car, bus and train wheels.

Then we get there and sit around for hours at a time.

If you are a hospital worker or gardener or construction worker, then you are fortunate because you are moving for a good part of your day.

But even if you move as part of your work, YOU STILL HAVE TO WALK as part of *The Great Australian Diet*.

This is the pathway to success.

# SBW - Strong is better than weak

Once you hit your 30s, muscle strength deteriorates at first slowly, then more and more rapidly. Most mature Westerners are WEAK.

Remember, there are approximately 600 muscles and about 180 joints in your body.

If the muscles are reasonably strong, it takes the strain off your joints and as well, you have more energy. Muscles also burn lots more calories than fat does – so having good muscles actually helps weight loss! You don't need huge muscles – just strong, well-toned muscles.

# Bottoms, arms and tummies – B.A.T. (Woman) – B.A.T. (Man)

My brother was watching Sue move her muscles and joints one day. My brother's name is Brian Arthur Tickell. He asked Sue if what she was doing would be good for him.

They both agreed that these exercises were **exactly** what he needed to firm up his butt and his arms and his tummy.

Brian decided that he could and should do them because they were so simple and easy. So Sue made a list of the exercises for Brian and we decided to name them in his honour!

.... the Brian Arthur Tickell exercises – B.A.T. exercises.

You are now being introduced to the **B.A.T.** exercises.

For **B.A.T. Women**, the

- **B** is **Bottoms**
- **A** is **Arms** and
- **T** is **Tummy**

Sue knows from first hand experience that huge improvements in muscle tone, strength, look and feel, can happen on the 91 DAY program. Regular muscle movement is the answer.

Breasts are close up on women's wish list, so we'll make that a separate category – **B** is also for **Boobs**.

Tight pectoral muscles (that sit under the breasts) are of great benefit here.

For **B.A.T. Men**, the

- **B** is **Butt**
- **A** is **Arms** and
- **T** is **Tummy**

Boobs are off the agenda for males, (though you wouldn't know it when you check out the local beach these days).

**T** is also for **Thighs** or quadriceps muscles.

If you wish to do a little more work on your thighs, climb some stairs most days or dust off the bicycle.

When we are in start-up mode during Week 1, do just one exercise set of six repetitions – no more.

If your muscles are really sore the next day, drop it back to four repetitions for a couple of days.

As the 91 DAYS go by, you gently increase repetitions and resistance, but DON'T overdo it. Remember that as the body matures, it takes a little longer for the recovery phase.

Exciting stuff!

The B.A.T. exercises are described and depicted in Part VI.

# OUMs - Other useful movements

Some people call these stretches, but I haven't got time to do half an hour of stretching because I'm a Type A person when I'm working.

Seriously, flexibility of body parts is really important, especially if you tend to get back pain and/or neck pain. A couple of minutes stretching and flexibility work can give you a huge pay-back.

My daughters, Anna and Amanda, have given us a list of OUMs. Anna and Amanda are both highly qualified physiotherapists.

The OUMs are desribed in Part VI.

Activity

# Coping >

Eating

# Coping

You must realise that you are not 'under stress'.

Stress is inside you.

Pressure is on the outside and stress is on the inside.

When a pressure is applied to the human body, the stress response can be positive or negative – your choice.

It all starts with attitude.

Your outlook on life, the way you react to different situations and the way you relate to people you love, like and don't particularly care for.

You have a choice as to whether you react positively or negatively to all the pressures in your life.

There is a third choice. No reaction at all ... just walk away.

Don't let anybody tell you that all stress is bad because it isn't.

There is **negative stress** which is the result of pressure you can't cope with and this leads to overload, exhaustion and burn out. And being around negative people doesn't help at all.

Then there is **positive stress**. This happens when you are feeling well, coping well and surrounding yourself with motivating thoughts and positive people.

Achievements result from positive stress responses.

It's very easy to lose perspective in times of extreme pressure.

Mountains can be made from molehills and minor problems can become insurmountable.

How well you cope with the different elements in your life can affect your physical and mental well-being … or is it the other way around?

Actually, it's both.

There are ways to improve how you cope with things. *The Great Australian Diet* will help you to improve your coping skills.

# Life skills

The three great life skills, or self-management skills, are **Activity** skills, **Coping** skills and **Eating** skills.

Coping skills are hugely important and of course good Activity and good Eating skills help us to cope much better.

Coping with life makes you younger and healthier.

How do I know that being in control, seeing the brighter side of things and laughing boosts the immune system? Well I just do.

Clever professors have measured antibody responses in people who have been thinking happy thoughts and then unpleasant thoughts and there is proof of a direct link between thought processes and the immune system.

If happy thoughts can have such an impact, imagine what a kiss or a hug from a loved one can do!

Kisses and hugs and watching movies about love also seem to increase the antibody response.

On the other hand, arguments and outpourings of sarcasm and nastiness have the reverse effect.

So there it is. Unhappy or depressed people have depressed immune systems.

But the opposite is true for loving, happy people. It was once believed that the immune system had a mind of its own.

Today, science has discovered that our immune system and our brain are closely connected by neurotransmission.

This is a science with a very long name – psychoneuroimmunology. If you can pronounce it, you're a genius.

What I am saying is that parts of the brain involved with emotion can affect not only our immune system, but our digestive system, our hearts, lungs and in fact most of our internal organs.

Being constantly negative, depressed, unhappy or just simply not coping can have a destructive effect on your body and it can also play havoc with your hormones. As you know well, when you are totally stressed out, your sex drive drops. You don't need a professor to tell you that.

So hugging is healthy and lack of hugging is probably damaging to your health.

Touch deprivation among pre-school children has a significant downside. Kids who are separated from their mothers experience a higher frequency of illness.

The immune system boost is obvious when the bond between mother and baby is strong. Breast feeding is an enormous start to life for infants.

Then, of course, there is a thing called **stress** – a great destroyer of the immune system.

What is stress anyway?

Stress is the body's reaction to an outside pressure.

You can't be 'under stress' because there's no stress out there to be under. Stress is an internal phenomenon.

So when you apply the same pressure to a group of individuals – sit back and watch what happens.

Different stress responses come from different people.

It is the person's perception of and attitude towards this pressure that determines the body's reaction.

> Example 1: **Person cuts you off in traffic**

*Reaction A*

Scream. Go red in face. Blood pressure up. Heart racing. Chase other car. Make rude gestures. ISA gonna kill him! **ISA** is Inside Aggression – the muscle around your heart arteries can clamp down – can bring on heart attack – can kill you.

*Reaction B*

Smile. That person will kill himself/herself one day. That's their problem. That's life.

> Example 2: **You have a problem, a big problem**

*Reaction A*

This is hopeless. I'll never work it out. This is too big for me. Panic, corridor thinking. More coffee, cigarettes, booze. Let's turn on the gas.

*Reaction B*

You think about it – you discuss it with others. You know from past experience there is always more than one way to solve a problem and often you don't see it straight away. You don't panic.

You achieve a reasonable outcome. You feel good. Makes you more confident about the next problem. That's life.

See? ... Same pressure – different stress responses.

## > Don't forget to take time out to smell the roses <

Laugh, touch, hug, give yourself mental rewards – read a great book, see a good movie, sit in a sunny garden and just daydream about pleasant things.

Get out of the pressure cooker and take a few days off every three or four months.

What about worry?

It can definitely pull your immune system down if you let it get on top of you. How do you deal with worries?

Take a blank page and draw a line down the middle. On the left side you write CAN DO and on the right side you write CAN'T DO.

Now what are you worried about?

*'Umm ... the cyclone.'*

What cyclone?

*'The one off the coast – there is a 20% chance it will hit the mainland.'*

Can you do anything about it?

*'All the contingency plans are in place. We've been through it before, and we're not leaving town.'*

So there's nothing else you can do?

*'No.'*

Right, well let's put that one under CAN'T DO.

What else are you worried about?

*'The mother-in-law, I worry about the mother-in-law.'*

Can you do anything but worry about her?

*'Well, I guess I could leave home … I guess I could … no … I guess not.'*

That's another one for the CAN'T DO column.

You see, you can get by with mothers-in-law, you can co-exist with them. You can co-exist with a lot of pressures.

One of the great things about the brain (which itself is like a pressure cooker) is that it has little compartments.

You can put a worry that you can't do anything about in one of the little boxes and lock it up so it doesn't bother you except when you let it out.

Why don't you set aside 20 minutes every couple of days when you just worry, worry, worry about these little things and then lock them up again?

The clever people don't worry all day about these stupid things, but the worriers have the page full up in the CAN'T DO column and they have only one, two or three things in the CAN DO column.

Why are you wasting so much of your life? It's dribbling away.

You are worrying about things you cannot control or affect. Stick them in compartments or forget them all together. If you don't, they'll get to you and completely destroy your life.

Life is for living.

What about the CAN DOs?

Do them.

Get a management plan, get an action plan going.

You can definitely help people sort things out. Take another blank page and draw a horizontal line across the middle of the page. We'll call it the thinking line. Which side of that line takes most of your time – above the line or below the line?

Now when your business encounters a hiccup or your cat dies, there is worry or grief and you get a little down. Your spirits go down, your attitude goes down ... normal human emotions ... grief, depression, anxiety, self-pity ... AND YOU DIVE UNDER THE LINE.

How long are you going to stay down there if your cat dies? An hour, a day, three weeks, three months? You see most winners come up again relatively quickly – they spend 70 or 80 percent plus of their time thinking above the line.

Then again, I don't believe it's good to spend 100 percent of your thinking time way up there. If you laugh non-stop, someone will lock you up. Everything moves in cycles, and the contrast between down and up is rewarding.

Some people worry if they've got nothing to worry about! They would rather have a bit of pressure, a problem to work on. The wheels are going to fall off most things some of the time, and they do, and that's good because it's the pressure, the stimulus, to turn things around.

It is frightening that your greatest asset, your mind, can turn on you and destroy you. But only if you let it.

Keep those ridiculous worries locked up in the little boxes over on the side and let them out for a breather just now and then.

## Behaviour Types

Broadly speaking, people fit into three behaviour types.

### *Type A*

Type A people are generally ambitious, fast moving creatures who are usually poor listeners and therefore tend to interrupt others.

Type As hate queues and red traffic lights, they tap their pen on the table, they tap their foot on the floor and male Type As usually push the flush button on the toilet before they've finished peeing.

### *Type B*

Type B people are laid back, are good listeners and have patience. They don't earn as much money, but they live a long time!

Material things and counting to achieve are far less important to Type B people.

### *Type C*

Type C people internalise pressures, fears, jealousies, problems and don't get things off their chest.

Type As, especially the aggressive Type As are more prone to heart attacks.

Type Cs seem to run higher risks for internal diseases such as cancer.

Type Bs probably have lower risks of developing any disease.

The best behaviour or personality 'Type' is probably B or AB. An AB is an A Type at work but this person can easily 'switch off' on a regular basis.

Where do you think you fit in?

# Taking the 'f' out of life

If you take the 'f' out of life, you are living a lie, and that's the truth. There are millions of people out there living a lie, because the relevant 'f' things have disappeared.

So if you had the next three months off with no work, no stress, no money worries, no time pressures, what things beginning with 'f' would you put back into your life to make it a *real life* instead of a lie?

I can hear you already, muttering some 'f' words I don't want to know about, but I'll give you a summary of the thousands of responses I have to this question from people all over the world.

## > No. 1 is Family

People would put more family back into their life – it's the biggest single support system available to the human body and yes, isn't it sad when you consider how many families fall to pieces? Go on, phone your brother – the one you haven't spoken to for years.

Go and have a beer or a glass of wine together and give him a huge hug and a slap on the back – OK?

## > No. 2 is Fun

Yes, fun. So many people these days take themselves soooo seriously and of course they don't have time for fun. Laughter is the best medicine, no doubt about it.

**Having fun, like being happy, is a daily decision**

## No. 3 is Friendships

'*But I've got friends*' you say. Yes, but do you have friendships with your friends? When was the last time you actually did something together and gave up some time to have a good chat or maybe ask for their opinion or a little advice about a problem?

## No. 4 is Faith

I am not talking about religion here, I'm talking about a thing that smacks you in the face when you discover what goes on in the lives of long-living people – the people the diet gurus have never been to visit. It's a 'thing' called spirituality.

What is spirituality? It is a belief in something bigger than yourself. It is a reason to exist. It also involves a sense of 'fair play' – win/win situations rather than '*I win, you lose*'.

Here are two statements to think about.

- Spiritual people are happy and contented.
- People who commit suicide do not have spirituality as part of their lives.

These four 'f' words are so important. We need to constantly remind ourselves of the power these words play in the game of life. *The Great Australian Diet* puts the 'f' back into life.

# The four aces

Life is like a game of cards and you cannot be truly happy unless you hold all Four Aces.

Let me introduce you to **my** pack of cards.

There is the *Ace of Diamonds*. This represents the drive for wealth … show me the money.

If that's the only ace in your pack, you won't find happiness. Western life is a counting, game, isn't it? It's count, count, count. Money, money, money. But you show me a person with the diamonds and a heap of money and I can show you plenty of miserable people, whether they're multi-millionaires or billionaires.

Money doesn't make you happy. You can buy friends, and you can rent a few friends for a while, but unless you've got the other three Aces in your pack, you haven't got a complete life. You can't be happy, truly happy, without all the four Aces.

Then there is the *Ace of Hearts*. This represents relationships, family, spirituality, belief systems and compassion.

If this is the one ace you **don't hold**, you won't find happiness. Show me the guy with the diamonds and no heart and I'll show you one empty person.

Then there are the other two Aces in the pack you need to complete the happiness circle – the *Ace of Spades* and the *Ace of Clubs*.

The Spade represents your work ethic. We all need to do some digging, we need to 'get our hands dirty' and 'do the hard yards'.

The more you work at something, the better you should be getting. If you're not getting better, seek help. Maybe a coach.

And remember, if you get something easily, it doesn't mean as much. Everyone seems to want things too easily. We have to keep up with the Jones's – a TV in every room, three cars in the garage.

People have to understand that anything you get too easily definitely doesn't mean as much. So you win the lottery – that's easy money.

You party on and in a year's time most of it has disappeared, or you've invested badly.

And what about the *Ace of Clubs*? This card represents social contact. People forget their mates, they really do. Do you have any friends? *Oh, yes*. When did you last go down to the club and have a beer or a cocktail and just sit around and have a yarn? *Oh, I can't remember*.

Well, isn't that sad?

It's sad. You need your mates. Have a drink, tell a story, all that sort of stuff. And don't forget the Joker in your pack. See the funny side of life.

Have a laugh. It's great medicine.

If you hold the Four Aces in your pack of cards, you can be truly happy. After all, what's the ultimate aim in life?

**Happiness**.

# Hakuna Matata

My son and his partner have just completed an amazing trip.

They travelled from Australia, through various mid-Asian countries on the way to China, India and some Russian Provinces and then their aim was to go overland all the way from Cairo to Capetown. They made it.

David is a Medical Doctor and will soon be a Paediatrician, looking after unwell little kids. David didn't stay in many hotels at all, but rather stayed in villages and with families in their homes. He watched and listened and learnt the local customs. He discovered all over again that the way to live a long, healthy and happy life is to steer away from the Western 'civilised' way of eating.

So much for **diet books** that tell us to eat heaps of fat.

David told me that in some African countries Swahili is still the major language.

Have you seen *The Lion King*? If you haven't – please do.

Fantastic music came out of that movie and one of the best sayings of all time. HAKUNA MATATA – it means '*No worries*' in Swahili. From now on, if you are having a bad day, hum the music – learn the song – sing the song. Remember, there are many people worse off than you.

If you are having a **really** bad day, go visit the Cancer Ward at the nearest Children's Hospital.

Now, who's having the bad day ...?

Are you with me?

Activity

Coping

# Eating >

# Eating

You are what you eat.

Never has there been a more true saying.

*The Great Australian Diet: The Atkins Alternative* will arm you with the knowledge and the inspiration to eat good foods, and achieve healthy **and** long-term weight loss. It's not rocket science and you don't need to carry a calculator or carb counter or charts with all sorts of numbers. All you need is some clear thinking. That's right. I'll give you the simple information about what is real and what is not so real.

These are the principles of *The Great Australian Diet*.

They are so simple and easy to put into practice. I could never have come across these principles just sitting in an office. It is really obvious that lean, energetic healthy people live their lives this way.

THAT'S WHY WE NEED AN ALTERNATIVE.

Swing the pendulum the alternate way and reap the benefits.

# Basic and Bonus

There are two food groups in the world.

Some nutritionists say there are four food groups and others say there are five food groups, but I say there are two food groups and I am right because I've been in marketing and I know about the KISS principle (Keep It Simple Stupid).

One food group is called BASIC and the other food group is called BONUS. Basic Foods are Plant Foods – vegetables, fruits, grains, grain breads, *less refined* pastas and rice, and don't forget nuts and seeds – not lots, just a few.

If you live on these to the exclusion of all else, then you are a fanatic.

You tend to run out of friends, you never get invited out to dinner and you are in danger of becoming a social outcast.

The great thing about my program is that I really don't care what you eat. You can actually eat anything you like and you can even eat Bonus Foods.

What's a Bonus Food? A Bonus Food is everything that is not a Basic Food, which makes it very easy to work out. Red meat, cheese, ice cream, chocolates, puddings, etc. etc. Great aren't they?

I don't care if you eat them – the critical thing is BALANCE. Where is the balance? Where is the pendulum?

Think of your eating choices as a swinging pendulum – BASIC on one side and BONUS on the other side.

The wonderful thing about *The Great Australian Diet* is that after two or three weeks, you don't actually want to eat BONUS Foods much at all – just now and then.

If you are a Western-style eater, your pendulum is most likely way over there on the Bonus side.

But isn't red meat good for you?

Of course it is. It has protein, high-quality protein – it has iron – it has vitamin B12 which is difficult to come by in other foods.

Why don't you have some every now and again? Maybe once a week or maybe twice a week or maybe three serves a week, but you wouldn't go past three times a week if you were half smart.

Now you're going to tell me about your dear old granddad down on the farm who had bacon and eggs for breakfast, sausages for lunch and steak for dinner and then some supper as well. That's three or four times a day he ate meat and he died when he was 99. So what about that?

I guarantee one thing about your granddad – he was physically working 14 hours a day and you don't. It's very hard to get away with that sort of eating if you just sit on your butt. And, besides, the exception doesn't prove the general rule.

What about huge lumps of cheese, full of saturated animal fat that may stick to the inside of your arteries?

Sure, eat a little cheese here and there, but why do you need to go past that? A little grated cheese on the salad or minestrone is fine, but do you need to eat huge mouthfuls of the stuff? That's Bonus, not Basic.

The best way to eat less animal fat is to visualise the fat actually sludging up your tiny, tiny coronary arteries – the arteries that keep your heart alive.

The *largest* of the coronary arteries is one-fifth the width of your little finger. Not very big, eh? These arteries have already gathered some sludge, **so there's not much room in there**.

Chocolates? Fine as a treat just now and then.

Remember, **Basic is Plant and Bonus is not Plant**. Sure, eat some Bonus Food, but here comes the Two-thirds, One-third deal.

The greatest rule of nutrition ever invented is this (and I invented it). It's the Two-thirds, One-third rule.

# Two-thirds, One-third

If you are prepared to eat at least two-thirds of the food that you put in your face as Plant Food, and if you are prepared to eat only one-third or less as flesh food and other food, then that's all you need to know.

You can virtually forget all the other stuff you've heard about fat and cholesterol, if you want to, because there is no cholesterol (nil, nought, zero) in any Plant Food and very little fat in Plant Food, except in olives and avocados. And by the way, the fat in the latter two is monounsaturated fat or Mediterranean fat, which is the best type of fat around.

Maybe you will go into a hotel or restaurant tonight and tell the waiter that Dr John said you can have a Bonus, so you order steak.

*'A steak please, medium rare, nice and juicy.'*

So here comes the plate and here's the steak hanging over the sides of the plate and here are a few peas, two sticks of asparagus and probably some fries. You see, the restaurant stuffed up the rule, didn't they?

They gave you 2/3 or more flesh, and 1/3 or less plant, and lots of people leave the plant anyway.

What about the Eastern Culture?

Here's the plate, here's the rice, here are the vegetables all over the place. Then they have small portions of protein – meat, fish, chicken.

They've got the rule right – 2/3 plant, 1/3 flesh.

*'Now wait just a minute, how come we are living till 80, 85 years of age at this stage if we eat all this crappy food?'*

I'll tell you how come.

First, we dramatically reduced childbirth deaths – women rarely die having babies nowadays – and then we got rid of infectious diseases – the typhoid, the cholera – and nobody tends to die now of tuberculosis or polio in Western countries. So that moved us back to three score years and ten, and then we added another eight, ten, 12 years.

How did we do that? Medical technology – absolutely brilliant medical technology – unaffordable, but brilliant. Stents, balloons, drugs costing billions of dollars each day.

We're living longer, but we're getting sicker earlier. Instead of presenting with heart disease, cancer, arthritis and diabetes in our 80s, they're happening in our 50s, 40s and even 30s!!!

I'm telling you the best way to eat is the 2/3, 1/3 way.

What about eating out? The chef generally does a superb job and then often covers the masterpiece with gravy or sauces.

You may say, '*But I love the gravy and sauces*'. So you are immediately doubling the calories. Why don't you order the sauce on the side or in little crock pots because you only need an eighth of the sauce for the same taste? – What a great idea!

Don't allow oil or dressing to be poured all over the salad. Order it on the side, because again you only need a sixth or an eighth of the oil or dressing for the same taste.

You need to become a little assertive when you walk into a restaurant. You can have two appetisers if you want – a seafood appetiser then perhaps a pasta appetiser. They say, *'Oh, you're not allowed to do that'*. So you run right through the menu to please the restaurateur. If you choose to, you can order an appetiser and then a plate of roasted vegetables.

They usually think you are crazy and they look at you and they point at you and all that.

If they do prepare the vegetable platter and want to impress you and retain your custom, they will do a superb vegetable platter, and at the end of the night, have no idea how much to charge you!

Vegetable Platter – usually half the price of a main course. You save money and your life as well.

Or try another trick – order some roasted vegetables as an appetiser! You can be nicely assertive in restaurants. You don't need to be rude, just nicely assertive.

What I want to get through to you is this – the body's desire for food is pretty simple. One of the great differences between chronically overweight people and those that are not ...

For the overweight, food generally is THE MAIN EVENT or at least A MAIN EVENT, while for others, food is what you eat when you are hungry.

# The amazing Rule of 15

My message is simple. The greater the range of Plant Foods you eat every day and the more colours you eat, the stronger your immune system will be.

At this stage of my medical career, I've given up sitting behind a desk handing out Valium. Instead I travel, I speak at meetings and company conferences, I go to different countries and I watch what people eat and what diseases they get.

I am absolutely convinced that if you wish to reduce your risk of preventable cancers such as breast, bowel, prostate and lung cancer by up to 75%, then you should aim to eat 15 different Plant Foods every day – different varieties, different colours, small portions of vegetables, fruits, nuts, grains and seeds.

The **Rule of 15** also plays a major role in *The Great Australian Diet* program.

*'You're crazy. I could never eat 15 a day.'*

Yes you can. Make it a game and at least get close to the 15. If my kids can play the game, so can you.

If you stayed in a hotel last night I guarantee this morning there were ten or 12 different fruits sitting on the breakfast buffet.

But people are boring – they only choose two. Even at home – four, five or six is easy. Have a plate of various sliced fruits sitting in the fridge.

Lunch – Go down to the salad bar and have six or seven different things in your grain-bread sandwich, or if it's self-serve, on your plate.

Dinner – Fish or meat and two vegetables. Why not six vegetables? It's no trouble. (Grandma always cooked six vegetables.)

# H.I. Index – Human Interference

So what is this H.I. Index?

It is the measure of Human Interference – in other words, how much or how badly humans have interfered with your food.

Another way of looking at this is how natural is your food – is it as nature intended?

You could draw a line down the middle of a page and to the left you could have the heading ... 'Before picked or killed' and to the right of the page ... 'After picked or killed'.

The obvious 'Befores' would include things like feed (added antibiotics, steroids) spraying, genetic modification, other growth factors etc., and there are a million 'Afters' such as storage, chemical additives, preservatives, colourings, canning, packaging (frozen is fine), salting, sugaring, adding to, subtracting from, refining, processing, squashing, peeling, and a big one of course is the mode of cooking, especially deep frying.

The H.I. Index is a lot better than the G.I. Index because the G.I. Index scares people and they stop eating many of the wonderful real foods, just because of a number they read in a book.

Okinawan Elders don't go to supermarkets – they go to real markets and they don't need to learn how to read labels because there are no labels on the vegetables and fruits and fish and meats they consume, nor on the jasmine and green teas they drink every day.

How about an example?

I'll do better than that. Later on in this book I will give you lots of examples in the Chapter titled 'THINK AND WIN'.

# High protein, high fat – way to go?

Every decade or so, the high protein, high fat diet surfaces again. Of course it works and produces weight loss – any disciplined eating plan works and you lose weight.

Question: Do you lose weight short-term or long-term?

Now, when you read a diet book, ask yourself this – has the author ever been to a country where there are no fat people and watched what they eat?

As I've said before, the diet gurus write diet books that are 500 pages long – 498 pages on what to eat, one page on exercise and one page on stress. Then they put disclaimers all over the diet saying maybe you shouldn't do this if you are pregnant or have heart disease or diabetes or kidney disease or if you are on medication or you got out on the wrong side of bed! And you should check with your doctor before you take a walk.

Do Asian villagers check with their doctor before they eat their vegetables and rice and walk through the hills and valleys?

No they don't.

This could be a good way to work out if a 'diet' is any good. If the disclaimer starts excluding various people with various ailments and pregnant women, then maybe the diet is dangerous?

(Pregnancy is a normal part of life – right now, today, there are millions of pregnant women in the world. Why should they be excluded if the program is safe?)

So let's go and look at the long-living races of people who are normal weight – are lean and energetic – have no retirement homes or coronary care wards – enjoy a very low risk of cancer and are **happy**.

What do they eat? A huge range of Plant Foods, some protein and little fat, NOT the other way around.

If you fall for the exact opposite trick what are you doing? In my opinion you are rapidly escalating your risk of various cancers and after all, isn't CANCER the scariest and most unwanted disease in Western 'civilized' countries?

And don't forget, the more protein and fat you push into your system, the more calcium is likely to leave your body as well.

The 'experts' who instruct you to cut out carbs are virtually telling you that these long-living, lean, happy people have no idea what they are doing.

So what's it to be – weight loss (and probably weight gain) with a constant overdose of high protein, high fat animal foods OR weight loss and weight control eating Plant Foods with millions of immune system boosting micro-nutrients?

We desperately need an ALTERNATIVE. *The Great Australian Diet* is the alternative for REAL LIFE.

Your call.

Part IV

# Fantastic information you can't live (well) without

# You can't live without blood pressure

Now we come to the heart of the matter and your blood pressure.

What is blood pressure anyway?

> **Blood pressure is very good because it keeps you alive. If you've got no blood pressure, you're dead**

Blood pressure is the pressure in an artery and it should be measured in an artery about the same level as your heart. So the blood pressure cuff is wrapped around your upper arm, where your biceps and triceps are, and this little cuff is pumped up until the pressure in the cuff is above the pressure in the artery.

Then you let the pressure out of the cuff and that's attached to a thing called a sphygmomanometer, which is an upright tube with numbers on it, and the tube contains mercury.

When the heart pumps, it pushes blood through the artery at a particular pressure. That's the top measurement of the blood pressure and it's called the systolic blood pressure.

The doctor or the nurse applies a stethoscope to your artery just below the cuff and as the pressure of the cuff is gradually reduced, they can hear the blood start to pump.

So as soon as that blood comes through, that's the pressure in the artery, the systolic pressure, which equates to the pressure when the heart is pumping.

Now, the heart pumps somewhere between 50 and 100 times a minute, and that's another story, because if the heart is pumping less times per minute, it usually means you're fitter.

And when your heart is fitter, it means it's more muscular and stronger and it can pump more blood per beat, which means it's more efficient.

So if your heart is pumping more slowly, when you expend energy and your heart rate fires up, you can produce more energy and you get less tired.

The fitter you are and the lower your resting heart rate, the more energy you have as the day goes on.

It's a simple thing that people don't understand. If you're sitting down and your heart is already banging away at 90 times a minute, you don't have much capacity to produce energy for long periods, so you become tired half way through the afternoon.

And people say, '*I'm getting old*'. It has nothing to do with you getting old. Your heart's just not strong enough.

'*How do I get my heart strong?*'

We come back to movement again. You take your heart for a walk around the block, you cycle, swim, go to the gym and work out. Getting back to systolic pressure – it's the pressure in the artery when the heart's pumping.

When the heart relaxes between the pumps or the beats, the pressure drops. It doesn't drop to zero, it drops to what we call the diastolic level, which is a level lower than the systolic. And you can also hear that through the stethoscope. It's all to do with the ebb and flow of the blood going through the artery because of the heart's pumping action.

Generally speaking, if you are considered low risk, the blood pressure should be less than, say 140 the top one, and definitely less than 90 the bottom one. And every tick or point above those levels gives you a higher risk associated with heart disease, heart attack and stroke. Especially stroke.

So it's prudent to keep your blood pressure below 140 over 90. Of course, 130 over 85 is better and 115 over 75 is sensational. The best way to reduce blood pressure is to have fewer blood vessels for the heart to pump the blood through. And given that every few pounds of fat have miles of blood vessels in the fat, why would you be overweight and screw on miles and miles of extra pipes, putting the pressure up and making the pump work harder?

When we explain blood pressure in these simplistic terms, people start to understand and say, '*So I need a stronger pump.*'

How do you get one?

I repeat. You take your heart for a walk around the block, climb stairs, forget the valet parking and move at every opportunity.

And you say, '*I need fewer blood vessels, fewer pipes*'.

Correct.

How do you get fewer pipes? You reduce the amount of fat you carry. Muscle also contains a lot of pipes but that doesn't matter because the muscles are working tissue.

Muscles actually aid the flow of blood, whereas fat is totally inactive tissue and is resistant to the flow of blood. So if you have blood vessels in muscles, that's good, as long as you don't go crazy and pump your muscles to bulging status. If you have blood vessels in fat, that's resistance – not so good.

Get the weight off, lose those excess miles of blood vessels, tone up the 600 or so muscles in your body, and bring your blood pressure into the 'healthy' zone.

And let me tell you this. When you have achieved that transformation, you'll know all about it. You'll feel so good.

*The Great Australian Diet* will help you get that weight off – short-term and long-term.

# Cholesterol made simple

This is a very technical subject but there is so much written about it and spoken about it, you may as well have some information so you can nod your head and look really wise when it comes up in conversation.

Cholesterol is a chemical substance used in the body for many and various things. One is to assist in the metabolism of fats. It also aids in the production of hormones, especially the sex hormones and cholesterol helps maintain the health of nerve sheaths.

So we need cholesterol. If you don't have any cholesterol, you're not alive. The body actually manufactures around three-quarters of the cholesterol in your system. So we eat cholesterol and we also produce cholesterol in our liver.

The body is very clever at working out how much cholesterol it needs. The more animal fat you eat, the more your liver can be stimulated to produce cholesterol.

The amount of cholesterol you eat is possibly not as relevant as the quantity of saturated fat or animal fat you eat – got that? If you're walking up and down the supermarket aisles and you see a product with 'no cholesterol' or 'low cholesterol', take little notice.

Search further and see how much animal fat, or saturated fat, is in the product.

Interesting – if you take a vegetarian, a vegan, eating vegetables only, Plant Foods only, and tip cholesterol into them via, say, egg yolks and prawns, the blood cholesterol level hardly moves.

But if you take a person who is indulging in excess animal foods and processed foods, thereby creating a heavy intake of saturated fat, and then pour cholesterol into them, the blood cholesterol level seems to move upwards.

So maybe it's not the ingestion of cholesterol *per se* that seems to affect your blood cholesterol levels. I believe it is more dependent on the ingestion of animal fat.

Science is telling us that a meal high in animal fat is likely to cause immediate changes inside arteries that can lead to spasm, narrowing of the blood vessels, blood clotting and may even bring on a heart attack. **If somebody is telling you to eat more high fat meals, then personally, I'd be worried.**

By the way, genetics do play a large part in determining what levels of cholesterol show up on your tests, so choosing your parents wisely is a factor.

Also, it's nice to know there are different types of cholesterol. Cholesterol is carried around the body by lipoproteins and the low density lipoproteins (LDLs) tend to dump cholesterol in the arteries. And you know what dumped cholesterol can do – stick to the inside of arteries and cause blockages. That's not good for blood flow and if the blood flow in the tiny coronary or heart arteries is limited, you're heading towards a heart attack or heart problem.

The high density lipoproteins (HDLs) tend to scavenge the cholesterol from arteries and transport it back to the liver where it's metabolised.

So the ratio of HDL to LDL is relevant. The more HDL, the better it is.

Let's say your cholesterol is 6. If your high-density fraction is greater than 25% of 6, or 1.5, then you have some measure of protection.

If your HDL is 2, and your total cholesterol is 6, that's an excellent level of protection. If your HDL is less than 25% – let's say your HDL is 1, and your total is 6 – then your risks of heart disease are likely to be a bit higher.

If your HDL is 0.5, which is only 1/12th of your cholesterol total, you could be heading for trouble. Can you increase the HDL fraction of the cholesterol high-density lipoproteins? The answer is yes.

Don't forget, cholesterol levels may be measured in two different units. If your cholesterol reading is in the hundreds, e.g. 180, 240, 310, etc then the multiplication or division factor is 38.61.

There are various things that the researchers say may help out here and exercise is one of them.

If you exercise, you increase your HDL levels and if you consume alcohol in *moderate* quantities this can, in some people, increase the 'good' cholesterol or HDL.

Other goodies in substances such as garlic and lecithin may help, but I guess mainstream medicos tend to dismiss those things as one-off 'magic bullets' or the 'answer under the rock' type of thing. Just because you eat garlic all day long doesn't mean you're going to live forever, but as I said, it may help.

It's a multiplicity of factors that affect these various measurements.

So cholesterol is good, cholesterol is bad. The higher the fraction of good cholesterol, or HDL, the more protection you have. You produce enough cholesterol to run your own body, therefore you don't need to consume much at all.

When we start explaining why the body was not built to eat a lot of animal fat, it becomes obvious that western people overindulge in animal foods. I'm not saying you shouldn't eat flesh, just take it easy.

My long living acquaintances in Okinawa are not vegetarians – they eat pork, but not much of it. They do however catch and eat a lot of fish.

**Carnivorous** beings eat flesh, meat. They rip flesh into lumps, they don't chew.

They swallow and what's digested is and the rest goes whoosh, out the back door. Short intestines.

**Herbivorous** beings eat plant.

Humans seem to be built as **Omnivorous** – able to deal with both. But take a peek at our teeth structure and the long, long length of our intestines and work it out for yourself. Too much flesh hanging around inside the bowel wall can cause problems.

Why is bowel cancer the No. 1 cancer in most 'civilized' Western countries?

I wonder?

And remember, there is **no** cholesterol in any Plant Food – nil, nought, zip, zero.

Don't forget that man was a hunter and would roam the plains looking for meat which was, by the way, lean and running meat – low saturated fat. It wasn't brought up in pens and coops and fed un-natural foods.

The meat was cooked and eaten there and then. It wasn't stored and eating meat was not an everyday occurrence because it wasn't caught every day.

Men were hunters of flesh foods and women were gatherers of plant foods. The anthropologists are telling us that women were probably better at gathering than men were at hunting.

Then somebody invented refrigeration. Bad move! This allowed us to keep flesh fresh (and eat it every day) and keep our sugary drinks cold so we could enjoy them to excess instead of drinking water.

Progress.

Really?

Animal fats are saturated fats. Do we need to give up eating meat altogether? I don't think so. I've just mentioned that the longest living race of people in the world eat some meat.

When refrigeration was invented, we started to eat meat every day.

That's what went wrong.

What about the other sorts of fats? Unsaturated fats tend to be more oils and liquids – they move, they go, whereas saturated fats tend to be more solid and they seem to stick.

The majority of vegetable oils and fish oils are unsaturated.

And the Mediterranean type of monounsaturated fats such as that in olives, olive oil and avocado are a relatively 'safe' form of fat.

The worst fats are the trans-fatty acids which happen especially in processed and manufactured foods.

They have been 'transformed' from their natural state by human intervention and they have been implicated in the increased risk of lots of diseases, including cancer.

If you read the packets, the products with the lowest levels of trans-fatty acids tell you on the label and those with high levels of the nasties don't want to mention it because they don't have to.

And which are the foods that have the highest level of disaster fats? You guessed it – donuts, muffins, cookies, pastries, fries, fried food – that kind of stuff.

What I'm saying here is that if you exercise regularly, cut back on your intake of animal fat and increase your fish and Plant Food intake, your cholesterol ratio will almost certainly improve and you can achieve healthy **and** sustained weight loss.

# Diabetes – do you want it?

If I were a statistician I could worry you a lot by telling you that the chance of your kids developing diabetes is now at the scary level – that's if they haven't got it already.

If your child has juvenile diabetes, then you probably know about it and more likely than not, you or they are already injecting insulin into their bodies day after day after day i.e. every day forever.

If you escape diabetes in your youth then you are now in line to suffer from all the negative effects of late-onset or Type II diabetes. 'Late-onset' is a misnomer because these days in the Western world it is not all that late when diabetes take a hold because we are being given our diagnosis fairly early in life ... 40s, 30s and even late 20s.

Diabetes of course affects blood vessels and heart attack risk, kidneys, eyesight – in fact most organs in the body. It can easily lead to premature death, i.e. it kills you if you don't look after it very carefully.

So what is diabetes?

The academics will start talking about the Islets of Langerhans in the Pancreas and all that stuff, but being really simple, the bottom line is this:

Your Pancreas sits in your middle region, just below the stomach.

When your body has a *sugar surge*, the Pancreas squirts out insulin to handle the rising sugar level in the blood and this helps metabolise the sugars into energy, water and other things.

With juvenile diabetes, kids are probably born without enough (or too much) fire power to produce the required quantities of insulin – there is a strong genetic influence here.

However, with late-onset diabetes, we generally do it to ourselves by wearing out our own insulin-producing ability – constantly bombarding the Pancreas with refined, processed foods and by not soaking up blood sugar levels by *moving* muscles.

There is an absolute correlation between lack of regular activity and Type II diabetes – no doubt about it.

It is truly amazing, the amount of time human beings take to plan various aspects of their lives.

You plan a holiday and once it is booked, you don't *ever* forget to take that holiday, do you? Why not?

Because you note it in your diary and mark out the days – that's why.

People regularly forget to go for a walk because it's not in their diary – that's why.

How many hours do you spend thinking about various investments and planning for the future? You may even have an investment adviser and you sit with this guy listening, planning, talking about real estate, the stock market, the forward building of assets – all that stuff.

I assume you would agree that health is your No. 1 asset?

No?

I'll tell you when you *will* agree ... when you haven't got your health. That's when you will agree with me 100%.

**They spend their health to get their wealth. And then with might and pain, they turn around and spend their wealth to get their health again**

That's if you don't drop dead first, which a mate of mine did last week – early 60s – sad.

How true is that statement about spending your health?

Walk away from diabetes.

Would you like to steer clear of being one of the millions of people in the civilized world who will become a DIABETIC in the next few months?

Easy.

## Walk away from it

If you are prepared to listen to your investment adviser (me) and walk for a half hour six days out of seven, your risk of developing diabetes plummets dramatically. And if you are prepared to listen to your investment adviser (me again) and eat mainly ***real foods*** i.e. with a low H.I. factor or Human Interference factor, then your risk of developing diabetes gets close to zero.

Good plan?

Takes a little time, takes a lot of thought, this investment business.

Even if you have Type II diabetes right now, you may be able to reduce or entirely dismiss your medication within a period of time. Discuss this with your Doctor, but why not start the investment plan first, then go and surprise him or her?

I get a good laugh out of the disclaimers on crazy diets. If the diet disclaimer says you shouldn't do this if you have kidney trouble or heart trouble or diabetes or you're pregnant or on medication or you got out on the wrong side of the bed, that says to me that the diet is *dangerous*. Here we go again.

Do Asian villagers check with their Doctor before they walk through the hills and valleys and do they check with their Doctor before they eat real vegetables and real grains and fruits and real fish and small amounts of real meat?

No. It's OK to take a walk.

## > Is your diet healthy or unhealthy?

A good way to check whether a diet is dangerous – read the fine print and if the disclaimer says things like those outlined above, then watch out!

It was recently pointed out to me by one of my colleagues that 'late-onset' diabetes or adult diabetes is also happening in children around middle to late puberty – big time. And of course, it is only prevalent in countries that have or are adopting the Western lifestyle.

Around 90% of 'your fault diabetes' is your own fault, but in the case of teenage children, who is to blame? Fairly obvious isn't it? ... Parents, processed food manufacturers, TV executives and educators who persist in destroying physical education as part of the process.

There is an epidemic happening out there and if the epidemic were a flu virus or cholera or typhoid affecting 20 million Americans and 150 million worldwide, people would be demanding action.

In the last two decades, diabetes numbers have doubled and in the next two, the disease will at least double or treble itself again.

The scariest thing is that up to half of the people with diabetes don't even know they've got it!

So the statistics I am quoting are only part of the equation.

But does it really matter?

I'll leave that up to you to work out, but to help out, here are a few notes.

> Diabetics have a far higher risk of the following problems ...

- high blood pressure
- blood clotting
- heart attacks
- strokes
- neuropathies including weakness, numbness and nerve pain
- impotence
- dementia
- infections of the lungs, urinary tract and skin
- cancer of various types
- hearing loss
- fractures
- depression

How are you feeling at this stage?

Are you still in the 'doesn't matter' group?

> The total community cost of diabetes in the US alone is billions of dollars every year.

> 90% of 'late-onset' diabetes cases are preventable

> The No.1 risk factor is obesity

One of the greatest challenges I see is the approach that health practitioners take when they are attempting to convince people out there to do something about it.

'Experts' say things like this:

'*Before starting exercise, individuals over 40 should take a stress test.*'

These peculiar directives have grown out of the fear of litigation by over-aggressive lawyers who throw lawsuits around like confetti.

There would be lines miles long outside every cardiologist's office in the country.

What's wrong with going for a half hour walk most days?

But the kids are the biggest worry.

What are we going to do about our fat kids?

Did you know that if you (parents) walk each day, the kids think that is **normal?** Did you know that if you (parents) sit on your backside all day, the kids think that is normal?

I looked inside a family fridge the other day, in a home I was visiting, to see if there was any real food. Well, there were cookies, brownies, TV dinners full of fat, three different types of ice cream and three **huge** plastic containers of fruit juice. What's wrong with eating an apple and drinking a glass of water?

That's too hard. Life is supposed to be easy.

Maybe **that's** the problem.

We're not prepared to work on it.

P.S. If you are concerned, or overweight or continually thirsty or running to the toilet or have a relative with diabetes, please go see your doctor for a little check up. OK?

# Superfoods

Is there such a thing as a super food? Browsing through magazines, one often comes across advertisements for extracts of something or other which could be 'the answer to life'.

My reading of the situation is this. Yes, there are super foods and no, there is not one particular super food. There is, as yet, no magic bullet – and there never will be.

If you eat right across the range of these foods, you're in business.

Of course, the big rage these days is for antioxidants, and with good reason. It seems that certain foods, or what's in them, can block the chemicals that may initiate cancer, and let me tell you this – cancer did not start last week or last month, but many years ago.

Most people develop rapidly dividing cells (mitotic cells) or precancerous cells quite commonly and it is up to your immune system to knock these over. If your immune system is not strong enough to wipe out these cells, this may be the start of a cancerous growth or tumour.

The ***antioxidants*** can snuff out oxygen free radicals, the nasties as we call them, and may even repair some of the cellular damage that has been done already. It is truly amazing that ordinary fruits and vegetables can be so effective against the carcinogens (cancer causing agents). Antioxidants include vitamin C, vitamin E and beta carotene for starters.

***Beta carotene***, the precursor of vitamin A or, if you like, the plant form of vitamin A, is high on the super antioxidant list and it comes in yellow, orange and deep greens such as *carrots, apricots, peaches, rock melons, sweet potatoes* and *spinach*.

Beta carotene is a carotenoid. Carotenoids are red and yellow plant pigments and the carotenoids are bioflavonoids. This really makes your head spin.

Bioflavonoids are a group of plant substances with recognised antioxidant properties and some ability to cut down inflammation of tissues. More about them in a minute.

Linus Pauling's old favourite ***Vitamin*** **C** is now a recognised antioxidant and of course vitamin C is abundant in *citrus fruits, strawberries* and *potatoes*.

***Vitamin*** **E**, another powerful antioxidant, is found in *nuts, grains, certain oils* and *leafy greens*. Is it just coincidental that heart disease really started to fire when breads became more and more refined, thus stuffing up the vitamin E content in the grains?

***Phytochemicals*** (means plant chemicals) are a buzz and stack up well in cruciferous vegetables as well as in *soybeans, onions* and *citrus fruit*. The *cruciferous vegetables* (so named because of the crucifix or cross-shaped arrangement of leaves or petals) are the *cabbage* family – *cabbage, cauliflower, brussels sprouts, broccoli, kale* and *bok choy*.

People say to me '*I don't like them*'. I say '*Well, get to like them. That's where all the micro nutrient action is.*'

It seems if you eat these day after day it is more difficult to happen upon breast cancer, colon cancer and others. But don't overcook them as you may destroy the indoles (whatever they are) – possibly the cancer crunchers.

*Tomatoes* have ***lycopene***, another antioxidant also found in *watermelons* and *apricots*. WOW! There is more available lycopene in cooked tomato (compared with raw) as well as tomato sauce and tomato paste.

Every male in the world should be eating tomato or tomato product every day – good for protection of the prostate gland. And don't forget, the lycopene is better absorbed in the presence of a little fat – make that olive oil as a first choice.

All ***green vegetables*** are full of antioxidants and the darker the green the more anti it is – the darker the better. Other carcinogen blockers (*pungent preventives*) come in *allium vegetables* such as garlic and onions.

***Garlic*** has long been considered an immune system booster – something to do with the sulphur compounds.

***Soybeans*** and ***soy products*** seem to play a part in the cancer prevention business, especially colon, breast and prostate cancers. Genistein is in the bean, the curd (tofu), soy milk and soy flour.

It is worth noting that the risk of developing hormone-dependent cancers in countries that consume high quantities of soy products and other flavonoid containing foods is dramatically lower than in Western countries.

Soy products include natural soybeans, tofu, miso paste and soup, soy milk, soy flour and roasted soybeans (soy nuts).

***Flavonoids*** are plant compounds found in soy products, *flaxseed, onions, cranberries, grapes, apples, broccoli* and some teas such as *jasmine tea.* Dried and canned *beans – chickpeas, lentils, kidney, pinto, navy, black, pink, white beans* – are also on the good guys' list.

***Soluble*** and ***insoluble fibre*** in various foods have been shown to be effective in lowering cholesterol levels (soluble fibre) and reducing the risk of colon cancer (insoluble fibre).

Soluble fibre is found in fruit, rice, and oat bran – insoluble fibre in peelings, whole grains, corn and many vegetables.

As we wander around the world, the peculiarities of the eating habits of certain races are noteworthy.

The Mediterranean reliance on ***monounsaturated fats*** such as *olive oil* is well documented. There is some protective influence against heart disease and cancer here.

The 'French paradox' is possibly a mystery – quite a deal of fatty food, but a surprisingly low incidence of heart disease. Perhaps it's not a mystery – the combination of *red wine* and love-making may do the trick!

Alcohol in moderation can raise the 'good' cholesterol fraction, and non-alcoholic chemicals like ***resveratrol*** may also help. This stuff also comes in *red grapes, purple grapes* and *dried raisins* that are not sundried.

***Quercetin*** is also in *red wine, red and yellow onions, broccoli* and *yellow squash.*

***Japanese green tea*** is a winner. For some reason, this tea seems to have antioxidant properties. And they regularly add the Jasmine flower to it.

The Eskimos are heavy on the ***Omega 3 oils*** which seem to do everything.

These oils come in *cold water fish*. Flaxseed and *flaxseed oil* are also heavy on Omega 3. They can thin the blood, lower cholesterol, reduce inflammation and may help reduce arthritic pain and asthmatic reactions.

They possibly reduce the risk of bowel cancer.

While we're on the subject of 'one thing does it all', aspirin is a blood thinner, an anti-inflammatory and may also reduce bowel cancer and breast cancer risk. Don't ask me how – nobody really knows. Just a small dose – a half or baby aspirin each day is enough. Be careful taking aspirin without your doctor's advice – it can irritate your stomach and make it bleed, and can affect your kidneys.

I know I've missed out on naming lots of miracle foods you've heard about, but this is a good sampling.

Notice how none of these super goodies are in meat or cheese, or fast foods? They mainly seem to hang around Plant Foods. Funny about that.

And Plant Foods are mainly carbohydrates!

# Nutritional supplements

To take or not to take additional vitamins and other supplements?

That is the question.

Conservative medical research has summarised the position by uttering statements such as this …

*'At present, no strong evidence can be found to support the routine preventive use of vitamins in well-nourished people.'*

What is a well-nourished person? The same one who works under incredible pressure, who misses out on the morning grains and fruit, who breathes toxic fumes from the city traffic and smokes stacks, who drinks coffee all day, who eats lots of fast foods, who drinks alcohol every day, and who does all the other things that lead to exceptional 'burn-up' of vitamins?

Vitamins and other micro-nutrients are substances which make the biochemical magic possible – producing energy and making body tissues, blood cells and hormones.

These nutrients are also necessary to maintain the immune system in tip-top shape, increasing resistance against infections and cancers.

What I'm saying is that stressful living and breathing rotten air use up large quantities of vitamins.

The bottom line is that go-go people who live and work in pressure-cooker environments need to eat very, very well, but usually they do just the opposite.

The medical profession has been slow to embrace the concept

of nutritional supplementation. Most doctors now prescribe vitamins for pregnant women, while some still say they are unnecessary (the vitamins, that is).

Don't dismiss the value of added nutrients as useless when the intake or absorption of food is less than perfect.

And don't forget many communities world-wide have embraced the use of herbal therapies for hundreds of years. So be careful if you quote some modern study (that lasted a few months) that says these therapies don't work. You might end up with egg on your face!

Had you asked me 20 years ago the question, '*Should I take nutritional supplements?*', I guess I would have said '*No*'.

Now science is moving towards the other side of the fence. There is strong evidence to suggest that the taking of nutritional supplements can pump up the immune system and increase resistance to various diseases, including cancers.

The antioxidant group can scavenge excess 'free' radicals, the nasty by-products of a metabolism under pressure.

Millions and millions of free radicals are produced by a body under pressure, a body that eats lousy food, is slobbish, inactive, worries too much, smokes, drinks lots of booze, and a body that generally cannot cope with the pressures of life.

Excess free radicals are also produced by bodies that exercise to excess, are very intense, and maybe don't sleep too well. Being aggressive and unfriendly doesn't help either.

If you have too many free radicals wandering around inside you, they stuff up your immune system and you are then more prone to colds, flu, cancers and illness in general.

Apart from that, you age faster than the calendar. Understand? You get older, quicker.

The human system actually needs a few free radicals but if there are too many, things go berserk.

I am convinced that the micro-nutrients act in concert, like an orchestra. If only the tuba player and the violinist show up, it doesn't sound so good, but if the whole orchestra is there, you have a top chance of a great performance, especially if the conductor is there as well.

So eat your vegetables, fruits, grains, nuts and seeds – the wider the variety, the better it is for you. And take some insurance as well.

## > Insurance

Whole of life insurance you get from an insurance salesperson means you have to live the whole of your life before you get the money. They only pay you when you're dead. There are forms of life insurance that provide a pay-off when you are alive. We've been talking about them.

Taking a walk. Improving muscle strength. Laughing. Eating great food. I consider that taking nutritional supplements is also good insurance – risk insurance.

I used to sit on the fence, but now I've jumped off the fence. I've been watching, listening, reading and researching the supplements business for more than 20 years.

What *do* I insure?

- I insure my car in case I have a crash.
- I insure my house just in case it burns down.

I do take supplements in case I don't do too well in the Activity, Coping and Eating departments.

I don't take overdoses of supplements because I know for sure that more is not better. Too much, too many, can have negative, even toxic effects and I worry about people who take large doses of supplements. Some people I know used to take so many pills, they rattled. Not any more – I've convinced them.

So do your homework and remember that highly trained athletes (where microseconds make a difference) have different needs compared with regular people who just want to be really healthy. Look for quality, reputation, excellence and a company prepared to be involved in ongoing research. Scientific validation is the name of the game these days. Most things can happen in the one pill and don't forget that women and men are different.

So yes, I do take an insurance policy every day. My insurance costs me less than a can of beer, a café latte or a couple of unnecessary calls from my mobile or cell phone.

# G.I. Blues

Elvis was right!

Long live the King … Elvis was way ahead of his time with the movie, *G.I. Blues*. He must have known that the world was going to be CONNED BY CARBS.

CARBS, low carbs, no carbs are the flavour of the moment. The hysteria surrounding the latest high fat, high protein diets are all about the damage that carbohydrates do to our systems.

**> Let's get one thing straight … vegetables and fruits are carbohydrates and they are the best two foods known to the human system <**

Once you start on an extended regimen of high fat/high protein eating, you are increasing the risk of the biggest disease problem in our Western society – CANCER.

You don't need to ask the scientists for their opinion on this one – just go to 100 different countries and keep your eyes open.

Cancer is the scariest disease on the agenda. Given the choice, people would rather have arthritis, diabetes and even heart disease before they would choose to have cancer. But this is not mentioned in the preamble to the hype associated with the usual diet plans.

G.I. is short for Glycaemic Index and this is a measure of the effect a particular food has on blood sugar levels. The higher the ranking of a food, the higher and more quickly the blood sugar rises.

Foods are rated on a scale relative to pure glucose which has a G.I. of 100. And yet, you read different books and different magazines, and they can't even agree on the rating of the same food! On one particular rating scale, banana has a G.I. of 60 and on another scale (diet book with 'Beach' in the title) banana is rated G.I. 89!

Another example: new potato – G.I. 54 as against new potato 101 in the other book.

The latter scale rates foods against white bread as the standard G.I. of 100 instead of glucose which they rank at G.I. 137. Talk about confusion!

I bumped into someone who refuses to eat pumpkin or watermelon because of their G.I. rating! How stupid … these are two of the best foods on earth, the former with heaps of beta carotene and the latter, lots of lycopene – both extremely valuable micro-nutrients. Another woman won't eat an apple or an orange (or vice-versa, I can't remember) because there's a seven point difference in the G.I. numbers – again, absolutely stupid.

Instead of looking at G.I. ratings, what we should be asking ourselves is this:

> *Is it a Plant Food, i.e. vegetable, fruit, grain, nut, seed?*

If the answer is YES, then that's GOOD – because Plant Food is Basic Food.

> *Have human beings got to this food (Plant Food or not Plant Food), and messed it up?* Have they refined it, processed it, peeled it, coloured it, smashed it, subtracted from it, added to it?

If the answer is NO, then that's really GOOD.

If it's only a little bit messed up, then that's NOT TOO BAD, but if it's messed up big time, then that's a PROBLEM.

If you eat crap food just now and then, good luck to you, but if you eat it most of the time, you have no respect for the greatest machine ever invented – YOU.

What these carb scaremongers don't bother to tell you is that you can easily reduce the overall G.I. rating of a mouthful of food (or a whole meal) by using a trick or two.

For example, add a little olive oil (as the Italians do with bruschetta) or some lemon juice. Add some soy foods to your meal or lentils, chickpeas and various types of beans. Grate a touch of cheese on the vegetable soup.

And 'they' tell us that you're not allowed to eat potato any more!

Well, I've figured that if the longest living race of people in the world eat sweet potato, it must be OK. Hey, it's not the potato, it's what you do to it and the quantity that makes the difference. We slice our potatoes into 20 or 30 pieces, dump them in animal fat and cover them with salt.

Westerners fill half their plate with chips or fries but they would never think of filling half their plate with broccoli or carrots.

By the way, sweet potato and even baked potato have a lower G.I. Index rating than carrots.

What about that, Mr Guru?

# Miki

I was having a pleasant conversation with a delightful 37-year-old lady who was born on the main island of Okinawa.

Let's call her Miki.

She was working as a guest relations person in a Western style hotel on the island and had previously studied in Canada and on the Japanese mainland.

Miki told me she was on a diet and I asked her why? She explained that she was overweight and needed to get back into shape.

I inquired as to what she meant by a diet and which foods she was and wasn't eating.

What came out of our discussion was the fact that she had gone back to eating the foods that her parents ate every day!

And yet the Western influence and the environment she had come home from had altered her normal eating and living patterns and changed her mode of thinking so that she considered she was actually dieting, when all she was doing was moving back to what she had grown up with.

Miki told me that her parents ate pork but very small portions. They ate fish most days, rice two or three times each day, many vegetables, soybeans and fruits.

Whilst living away from home she had found it increasingly difficult to eat Japanese village style and it was just easier to succumb to the Western routine.

So Miki's home-coming diet was to eat little red meat, more fish, vegetables and rice and to cut out refined junk and fries, as well as doing some walking and swimming each day.
Was it working?

But of course.

So, is this a diet or more of a reality check?

Your call.

# Kangaroo

Australia has the best red meat jumping around in its own big back yard.

- Very lean
- High iron content
- Low animal fat
- High PUFA

Not too sure about that PUFA claim?

Is that good?

Yes it is.

All four of the above are excellent positives. The kangaroo is a fast moving herbivore and obviously not fed anything artificial. No antibiotics, no growth factors, no nothing. It's all good.

Kangaroo meat is a fabulous source of protein, zinc and iron, and the iron comes in a form which is well absorbed by the human body. As you know, iron deficiency anaemia is common in women of childbearing ages, especially vegetarian females. How does a really good feed of meat sound and with only about two percent fat? That's right – 2%!

Tell me more ...

Now for the PUFAs.

These are the PolyUnsaturated Fatty Acids which can lead to lower cholesterol levels, reduced blood clotting and lower risk of heart attacks and stroke.

Kangaroo meat also has abundant levels of natural CLAs (Conjugated Linoleic Acids), which potentially have an association with a lower risk of some cancers, e.g. breast cancer. Previously, the highest known source of CLAs was dairy milk.

The bottom line?

If the kangaroo was sitting on the showroom floor and was lined up against beef and lamb, which one would you buy? The streamlined, jump-start kangaroo wins in virtually all departments and is definitely the sports model compared with the slower moving cow or sheep chassis.

But you don't fancy eating it, right?

Well, read on .... There are around 35 million kangaroos in Australia and they are a renewable natural resource – they are not going away. Five of the nearly 50 species are just fine for human consumption and the quality controls now in place are extremely strict.

Two million kangaroos are harvested each year as meat and who gets to eat most of it? Our pets.

Why should our domestic pets get all the breaks and have first call on this very healthy food? Not fair.

And where does the rest go? Most of it is exported for human consumption in Europe. What a pity.

They've jumped on the bandwagon and we are missing out.

So let's raise the bar a little higher. Kangaroo meat is gold medal material in the health stakes. Try some this week, and next week and the week after and you'll start to love it.

## > Kanga Tips

- Grill, stir-fry or BBQ
- Usually cheaper than beef or lamb
- Great flavour
- Must be cooked quickly because of its low fat content.

## > Tail Note

- Kangaroo meat can also assist in the prevention and management of diabetes.

Part V

# Really good ideas (R.G.I.s) and basic guidelines

>

# Really good ideas and basic guidelines

For the first 3 weeks, I'm going to advise you what to do.

Then after that, for the next 2 weeks, you're on your own.

Then in the following 3 weeks, I've got you again.

Then 2 weeks is yours, then the last 3 weeks, me.

OK?

Most diets begin on a Monday, but this is not like the other diets, so you can start any day you like.

But I'm the instructor, so let's start MONDAY.

Monday is DAY ONE.

For each of the three week periods when I'm calling the shots, we start with one or two days of CLEANSING. In the first week – two days of CLEANSING and in the second and third week – just one day of CLEANSING. This is not fasting, it's cleansing. I don't believe in fasting because you're liable to get hungry and hunger is not part of *The Great Australian Diet* 91 DAY deal.

And the great thing about this program is you *learn* about food.

*The Great Australian Diet* doesn't treat you like a dumbo. You start to get the hang of it and adjust your eating habits to fit in with the way you are feeling.

It's brilliant! It feels good!

If you want a piece of chocolate – OK – but why eat a giant chocolate muffin? There is no point in this huge muffin thing because you're only feeding your tongue. *You* don't want it – your taste buds do. The guys who make these calorie bombs should be run out of town.

Have one of my Fail-Safe Snacks instead (see Week 1 Day 2 in Part VII).

The Fail-Safe Snacks are fail-safe.

So here we go ...

We'll start with some **R.G.I.s (Really Good Ideas)** and **Basic Guidelines** just so we are beginning to think on the same wavelength.

# Really good ideas - (R.G.I.s)

It's a Really Good Idea to go to the market – not the supermarket. Take away the super and try the real market. They have fresh produce – great vegetables, fruits, fish, meats. These are the foods that humans haven't had the chance to mess around with. Real food, not plastic processed stuff.

The other worry with supermarkets is that as you approach the checkout chick, sorry, person, you are confronted by a tempting extravaganza of refined junk.

Don't eat huge meals. You just don't need them. Make sure you have a glass of water before you eat. A great way to fill yourself up before your main meal is to have a small bowl or cup of vegetable soup or miso soup.

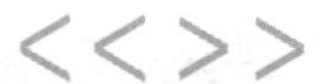

The best snacks are things that satisfy your tongue and your stomach, but have hardly any calories.

My favorites are a few sips of skim milk or soy milk and/or a couple of teaspoons of low fat yoghurt. I'm not a calorie counter but I can tell you that what I've just mentioned can be 10 or 20 calories, whilst just one bite of a chocolate or snack bar thing can be 100 or 200 calories and the whole chocolate bar up to 1000 calories. And while a small packet of chips is 500 to 600 calories, the big packs contain about 2500 calories. Wow! That's enough calories for more than a whole day!! You've got to be kidding.

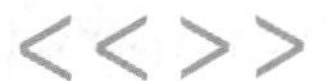

Drift toward foods that don't have labels. If you do read labels, they can frighten the living daylights out of you. For example vegetables and fruits don't have labels telling you what's in them, because you don't need to know. It's all good. Mind you, if they did have labels, it would say carbohydrates and sugar and then you probably wouldn't eat them.

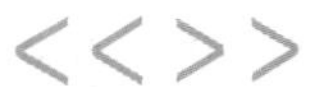

Fly to Asia and check into an Asian Hotel, not a Western Hotel, and go to breakfast next morning. A stunning array of fish, nuts, fruits, seeds, grains and soup awaits you. Now, that's the way to break your fast.

Variety is the name of the game. That's why the Rule of 15 works so well. It gives you more interest, more energy, more brain power. Don't forget that glucose feeds the brain. And of course if you do the Rule of 15, you have less risk of cancer.

<<>>

If you see a bunch of stairs, walk up them – feel your quads and your butt muscles contracting, tightening. Your thighs actually talk to each other and chat about what they've done today. Give them something good to talk about.

<<>>

You don't need to eat it all …

I was having coffee and a chat with my daughter the other day and as we were talking, she devoured a whole large muffin. I asked her why she ate the whole lot and she said, '*Because it's there*'.

I hate when people start sentences with *'In the old days …'* but here goes …

In the old days, we had nice little cup cakes but now we have gigantic muffins with choc chips or blueberries and a million calories. So leave half of it on the plate.

Did you know I'm one of the very few people in the world who can go to the mini-bar in a hotel room, grab a packet of potato crisps/chips, eat four and throw the rest in the bin or the trash?

*'But you've just wasted $3.'*

*'No, I've just saved my life'.*

<<>>

Struggling to reach THE RULE OF 15?

Think Minestrone.

<<>>

Hungry?

Think Minestrone.

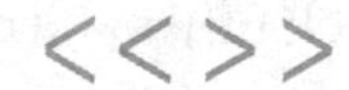

# Basic guidelines

It's the EXTRAS that are the biggest trap in the weight game. The snacks, the second helpings that you don't need, the 'health' bars, the packets of junk.

<<>>

Do you weigh yourself every day?

Well, don't.

Once a week is OK.

Every three weeks or so, check your dress size (girls too!). Try on this and that. Go the 91 DAYS, then re-assess your wardrobe.

## BBQs

Any good? Not too often. Once in a while is fine. Don't burn the flesh. When you burn and blacken flesh, you produce nitrosamines which can increase the risk of cancer.

## Alcohol

There are three levels of alcohol intake during the three weeks, depending on your level of desperation ...

- Not Desperate (N.D.) – don't drink any alcohol during the three weeks, or maybe a glass of wine at weekends.
- Moderately Desperate (M.D.) – one glass of wine with each evening meal on days 3, 4, 5, 6, 7.
- Definitely Desperate (D.D.) – one glass of wine days 3, 4, 5 and two glasses of wine on days 6 and 7.

A long time ago I invented AFDs. AFD means Alcohol Free Day.

The human machine works better with a regular touch of discipline.

## > Fruit Juice

Nutritious, but lots of calories. How many oranges do you need to squeeze to end up with a glass of orange juice? Four? Six? In the three week Switch On periods, no juice – eat the fruit instead.

## > Soft Drinks, Soda Pops

Why?

There are about three quarters of a billion soft drinks consumed in the US, EVERY DAY!

What's the point?

Billions of calories – that's the point.

What's wrong with water or a nice cup of tea?

## > Cereals

In the Switch On weeks, stay clear of cereals in packets, packages, boxes, cartons.

If you wish to re-introduce small helpings of whole grain cereals later on, then that's OK with me. A home-made muesli mix can be a good idea, but go easy on the serving size. Check out the recipe in the Recipe section.

## > Starch

Bread, potato and pasta are often referred to as 'starches' and are a no-no according to many diet books.

Starch is glucose, which is a pure form of energy and it burns 'clean'.

My belief is that it all has to do with the level of refinement, H.I. (human interference) and the quantity consumed.

Whole grain breads, real small potatoes, and a little pasta just now and then are all part of the game of life as played by many normal-weighted long-living people. Quantity is the problem.

## > Biscuits, Cookies

Humans have interfered. High H.I.

Only if you need a treat in the Hold weeks – it's your call.

## > Olive Oil

A teaspoon or two of the Mediterranean Magic doesn't go astray – it's clever – just a teaspoon is not many calories at all and it can make a major taste difference to quite a few foods.

## > Portions

When you eat meat, keep the size of the portion to 3 or 4 ounces (that's 90 to 120 grams).

**> Remember the Two-thirds, One-third rule <**

The steak is not supposed to overlap the whole plate, just one-third of the plate. The two-thirds is Plant Food – vegetables and salads.

## > Fast Food

Why do you need it? You don't. I would eat that stuff maybe three or four times a year – when I can't find anything else, like in an American Airport. And I only take a couple of bites then just throw the rest in the trash. Don't forget the human interference factor. Ask yourself – is it natural food or has someone messed it up?

## > Dressings

When you are served food in BONUS land, they say … '*What dressing do you want with that? Thousand Island, Blue Cheese, Ranch, etc.*'.

If I say, '*I don't want dressing, thank you*', they look at me with an inquisitive stare like I'm from Mars. So I say, '*I'll have it on the side, thanks*' – then that puts me in control.

You need about one eighth of the dressing for the same taste sensation. And you're saving another million calories and a ten mile walk.

## > Sauces

If a meal comes with a sauce, especially a cream based sauce or one you've never heard of, then I'll say it again – 'on the side'.

Remember, you only need a touch of sauce or gravy to satisfy your taste buds.

## > Water

'*Drink eight glasses of water a day*', they say.

'*You can't drink too much water*', they say.

Well, who are 'they'? – and I don't agree with them.

Whoever dreamed up this one was obviously on the crazy high protein/high fat deal because when you are eating mainly plant foods, you are taking in lots of water anyway (in the food). Vegetables and fruit are carbo***hydrates***. OK? If you are eating plenty of fruits and vegetables and having a glass of water before each meal, that's cool.

And, if it's hot or if you're thirsty or if you are doing heaps of exercise, take in some more.

By the way, unless you are exercising really hard for up to an hour or more, you don't need all those fancy sports drinks. Water is fine.

A good rule of thumb is this – if your urine is clear, your hydration is OK.

## > Spreads

Butter or margarine?

If it's a very thin scrape, who cares?

Actually I very rarely use either.

On my grain bread, my choices are usually 1. a thin spread of avocado, or 2. Tomato, or 3. a touch of olive oil and balsamic vinegar, or a combination of 1. and 2. or 2. and 3.

## > Sleep

Did you know that bad sleeping can be tied up with being overweight?

Well the scientists say it can.

Too little sleep can cause you to become a real mess. Too much sleep can turn you into a Dodo and lack of quality sleep is also a problem.

So how do you get a good night's sleep?

Here are some tricks.

- Maybe a nice glass of wine to settle you down.
- Physically tired people sleep better than mentally tired people.
- Try a relaxation technique – slow breathing is the beginning point. Buy a book and read all about it.
- Do some numbers in your head. Count backwards. Keep subtracting seven from 300.
- Close your eyes and think about wonderful things. Fantasise a little.

# Favourite foods

Here is a list of ten favourite foods that the longest living people in the world consume on a very regular basis –

- Rice
- Fish
- Soybeans
- Goya (bitter melon)
- Imo (sweet potato)
- Firm Tofu
- Miso Paste and Miso Soup
- Seaweed
- Shiitake Mushrooms
- Jasmine Tea

And guess what? The majority of these foods are full of carbohydrates!

Fish, soybeans and tofu are the richest sources of protein on this list.

By the way, how many out of these ten are regularly on your menu?

# Why would you eat these foods?

This chapter was going to be called 'Banned foods', but I don't ban foods so I have changed the name of this Chapter to 'Why would you eat these foods'?

Here are a few foods that you honestly don't need in the **Switch On** weeks – just don't go there.

- Croissants
- Commercial Muesli
- Cereals in a Box
- Fruit Juice
- Soft Drinks, Soda Pops
- Muffins
- Donuts
- Reheated Foods
- Chicken (except skinless breast)
- White Bread
- Cookies, Biscuits
- Fast Foods
- Butter/Margarine
- Fries
- Fried Foods

- Snacks in Packets
- Dried Fruits
- Dressings (except a touch of olive oil or oil and vinegar)
- Sauces
- Luncheon Meats
- Pressed Meats
- Processed Meats
- Sausage
- 'Health' Bars

Part VI

# The Great Australian Diet: The complete 91 Day program

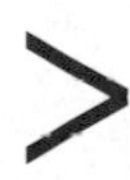

Switch On,

Then Hold,

Switch On,

Then Hold ...

**Switch On**, **then Hold** ... this is worth repeating.

Olympic athletes don't go full bore with their training all the time. Nobody in their right mind works seven days a week, every week of the year and every year till they die.

21 days at full pace is about as far as we can go with anything.

This is why *The Great Australian Diet* is so powerful. It works because we have our **Hold** times as well as our **Switch On** times.

You don't need to be a fanatic.

It's OK to have the occasional Bonus Food. It's OK not to exercise every day. **Switch On, then Hold** is designed to give you a bit of a break. I want you to think about what is good for you and then get into this moving thing regularly.

Think and be aware. Take the stairs next time instead of the elevator. Me? I get really excited these days when I see some stairs – my thighs are itching to climb them!

Go get the newspaper, but burn rubber now and then on the way. Your dog always wants to take a walk.

Become a kid again at the park – don't just watch your kids at play. Have a chat with your partner after dinner – while you take a stroll. 91 Days is all it takes. You'll love what happens to you because it becomes a part of you.

# The numbers game

I've decided we are going to work out how well you are doing with *The Great Australian Diet* by adding up numbers.

Is there another way?

You could email me a picture of your smiling face or send me some 'too big for me' clothing.

No. Let's stick with the numbers.

Every point you score is known as a Living*life* Point.

In this book you will find charts called the **91 Day Success Charts.** There are 13 of them, one for each week of the program. You can fill in these charts in your book or alternatively photocopy them and put them on the fridge or in your diary.

You must complete one chart by the end of each of the 13 weeks. **It is absolutely essential to do this during the Switch On weeks**.

If you don't do it in the **Hold** weeks, I will be disappointed.

Go on, do it anyway to see what happens when **you** are in the driver's seat.

There's no need to cheat because you're only fooling yourself.

The idea is to score around 72 Living*life* points during each **Switch On** week. In the **Hold** weeks, don't switch off – it's your call.

If you can still achieve close to 50 or 60 Living*life* points during the **Hold** weeks, I will be most pleased. *(So will you.)*

No questions at this stage, thank you.

Believe me, this works. Thousands of people have changed their lives for the better.

Trust me, I'm a Doctor.

But a *different* Doctor.

To my knowledge, this is the first program in the world that actually gives you points for hugging your kids and your loved ones.

You get points for laughing and points for having a good night's sleep. What's that got to do with losing weight, you ask me?

Everything!

Some of the other diet programs have never worked this out – they are too busy counting carbs!

# Activity >

Coping

Eating

Now we get down to business.

## > ACTIVITY IS THE A IN A C E <

- Burn Rubber
- SBWs – Strong is Better than Weak
    - B.A.T. Exercises
- OUMs – Other Useful Movements

The complete 91 DAY Activity Schedule is in Part VII.

There are three levels of activity to choose from

(a) Fanatical

(b) Moderate

(c) Zero (Slob)

Personally, I think (b) is a great choice.

I trust you choose (b) as well. If you choose (a), we'll see you at the Olympic Games. And if you are over the age of 35 and you choose (a), be very careful, because it might kill you. And, remember, fanatics are mostly boring.

**In the first 3 weeks of the program, you must move for at least 1% of each week!**

There are 168 hours in each week

so 1% = 1.68 hours …

that's 100 minutes.

What are you going to do for 100 minutes?

WALK!

No excuses.

# Burn rubber

Four days a week for 25 minutes (or five days a week for 20 minutes).

I don't mind which it is – it's your choice. *But when, what time? What shoes do I wear? What if it's raining/too cold/too hot/too windy/up hills/down hills?*

OK. OK.

This is how we'll handle it. I'll tell you what to do and you vary it if you need to.

Four days per week – 25 minute walk!

Saturday, Sunday and two weekdays.

Flat ground or gentle hills.

*How hard, how fast?*

Walk so that you are lightly puffing.

If you want to walk with someone else, that's fine.

If you prefer, do it by yourself – that's fine.

If you want to walk less than four days per week, forget it.

Go to the sports store and buy some proper walking shoes – comfortable, good support. If you buy good shoes they'll last you a long time.

For the best results you need to do weight-bearing exercise (i.e. walking) for at least 1% of your time during the first three weeks. No arguments here.

Other weight-bearing exercises include walking/jogging, running, stair climbing and bouncing on a mini-trampoline, but walking is fine by me.

If you want to do some non weight-bearing exercise such as cycling and swimming, then that's OK, but it **must** be **in addition** to the weight-bearing exercise.

Join a gym if you want, but that doesn't excuse you from the walking.

### > *What if I really can't walk?*

If you genuinely can't walk, what can you do that gets you moving and lightly puffing?

OK then, do it.

### > *Can I do more walking on the non-exercise day?*

If you wish, yes – but don't go crazy, and then all of a sudden, give up.

### > *What if I walk as part of my work?*

Great but you still must do 'lightly puffing' walking and SBWs and OUMs as part of the program.

### > *What if I'm too fit for this?*

Then jog if you want to, or combine walking and jogging, but don't go crazy. Nicely does it. I don't want you to harm yourself.

### > *No time?*

Honestly, that is the ***worst*** excuse I've ever heard. You're telling me you can't find 1% of your life to save your life ...!

# SBW - strong is better than weak

My lovely wife Sue became pregnant in her mid 40s (shock, horror) and gave birth to a bouncing baby boy to add to our collection of four older children.

A 14-year gap between child number four and child number five is not great for anyone's body, but turning a negative into a real positive, Sue used her skills as a Phys Ed Graduate and developed the simple B.A.T. exercises to tone, form and strengthen muscles in all the right places that people need – to look good and feel good.

As Sue says ...

*'I'm a busy person with five kids and if I can spend a few minutes four or five times a week doing the B.A.T. exercises, then so can you.'*

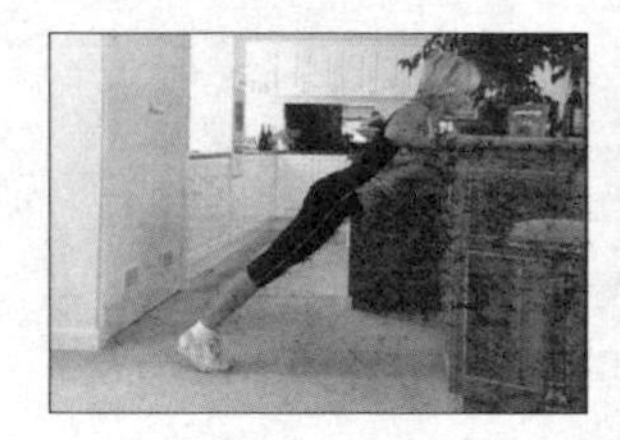
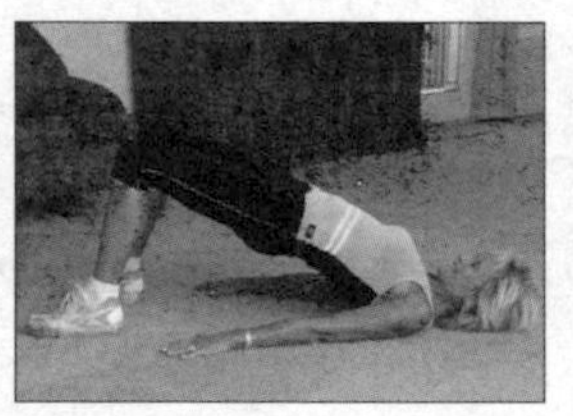
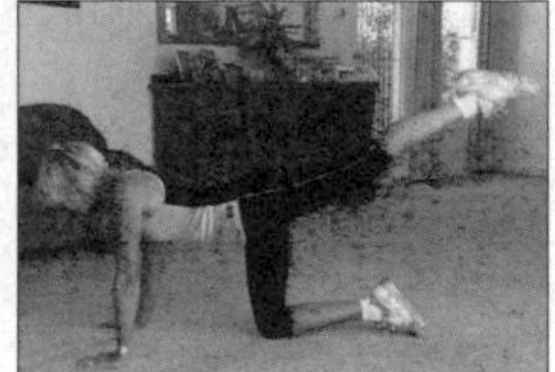

Sue - mid-50s - mother of five kids

Here's the plan for the SBWs.

| | Sets | Repetitions | Weight Women | Weight Men |
|---|---|---|---|---|
| WEEK 1 | 1 | 6 | 2 or 3 kg | 4 or 5 Kg |
| WEEK 2 | 1 | 8 | 2 or 3 Kg | 4 or 5 Kg |
| WEEK 3 | 1 | 10 | 2 or 3 Kg | 4 or 5 Kg |
| WEEK 4 – It 's up to you | | | | |
| WEEK 5 – It 's your call | | | | |
| If reasonably comfortable, move up a level | | | | |
| WEEK 6 | 2 | 6 | 2 or 3 Kg | 4 or 5 Kg |
| WEEK 7 | 2 | 8 | 2 or 3 Kg | 4 or 5 Kg |
| WEEK 8 | 2 | 10 | 2 or 3 Kg | 4 or 5 Kg |
| WEEK 9 – No worries! | | | | |
| WEEK 10 – Feeling good? | | | | |
| If reasonably comfortable, move up a level | | | | |
| WEEK 11 | 2 | 6 | 3 or 4 Kg | 5 or 6 Kg |
| WEEK 12 | 2 | 8 | 3 or 4 Kg | 5 or 6 Kg |
| WEEK 13 | 2 | 10 | 3 or 4 Kg | 5 or 6 Kg |

It's really easy. Don't worry about it now ... I'll add them to your day-by-day schedule – in Part VII.

You will need some hand-weights – some people call them dumb-bells – no idea why because it is a good idea to use them. Get the plastic covered ones – they look better and they don't rust.

**Women** – start with the 3 kg hand-weights.

Before you purchase the weights, pick them up and if they feel too heavy to use for regular exercises, then start with 2 kg weights.

**Men** – start with the 5 kg hand-weights.

Before you purchase the weights, pick them up and if they feel too heavy to use for regular exercises, then start with 4 kg weights.

# Bottoms, arms and tummies – B.A.T. (Woman) – B.A.T. (Man)

If Sue, a mature woman in her mid-50s (with five kids) can do this, so can you.

You want results?

You can have them.

Sue also underlines the fact that you can't 'spot' lose fat (i.e. lose fat from one particular area) with a weight loss regime. But you can certainly tighten and tone one particular 'spot' by regularly moving the muscles in that area.

Another challenge – if you starve yourself and lose lots of weight too quickly, it can make you look older, not younger, because your face can suffer with fast weight loss.

By the way, on your movement schedule chart, I've organised the **SBWs** and **OUMs** on the same day as your walk.

If you want to do these on different days, that's your call but you **MUST** do **4 WALKS**, **4 SBWs** and **4 OUMs** each week.

Otherwise, you don't score the necessary points and that would be a disaster.

## > B.A.T. exercises

These are the **B.A.T. Woman** and **B.A.T. Man** exercises ...

## > Bottom

### *Bridge*

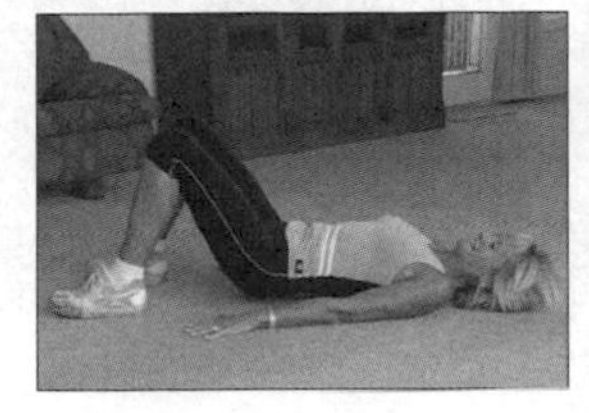
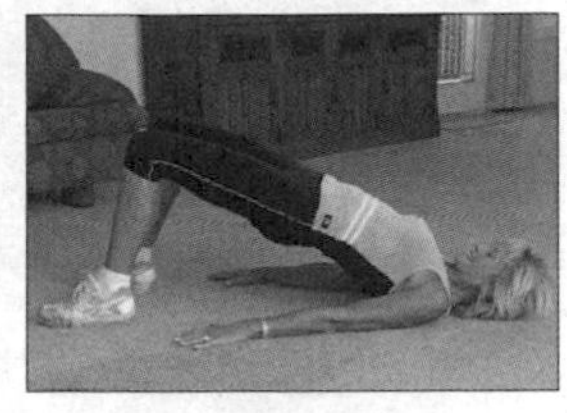

Lie on your back, knees bent, feet slightly apart and arms by your side. Push hips upward, tighten bottom. Hold for two to three seconds, then lower bottom back to the floor.

### *Side Leg Lifts*

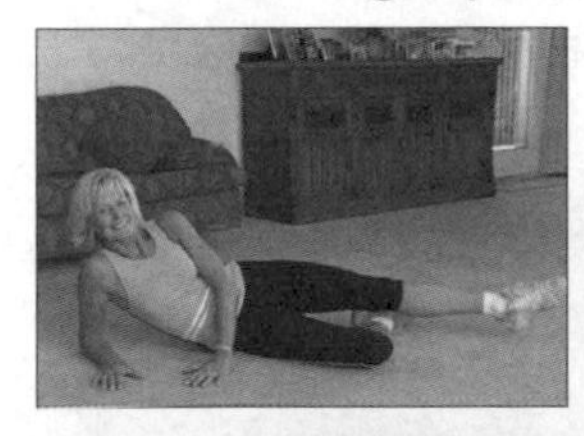
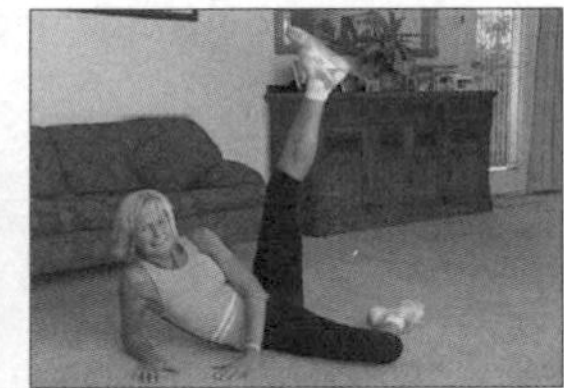
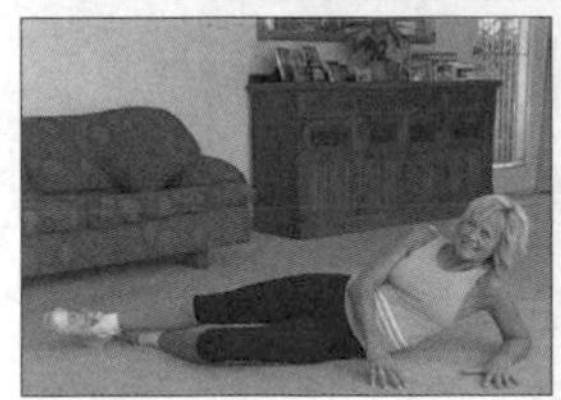
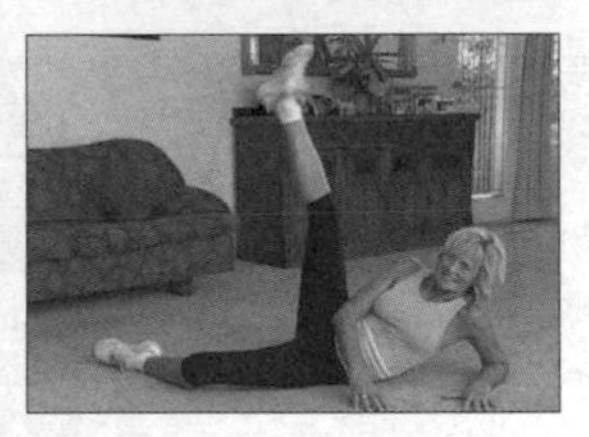

Lie on your left side, resting your body weight on your elbow. Bend your left leg to a comfortable angle and keep your right leg straight. Slowly raise your right leg to just above hip level. Gently return your right leg to the starting position. Repeat on the other side.

## *Leg Extensions*

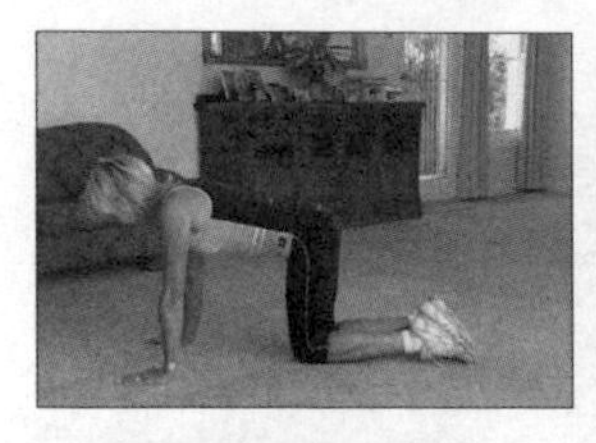
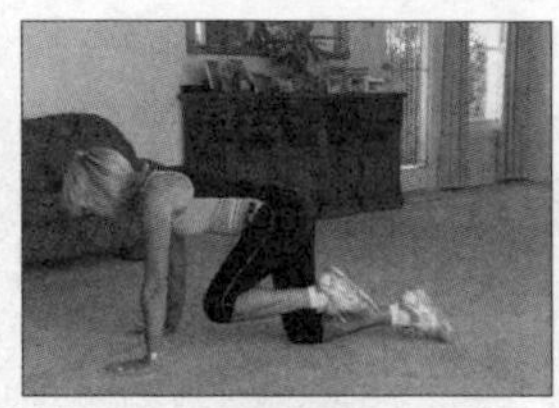
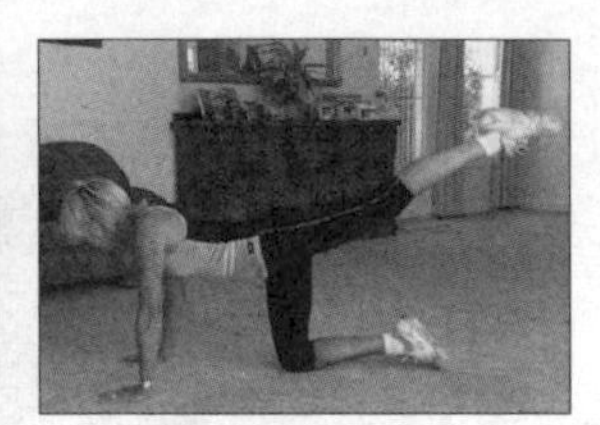
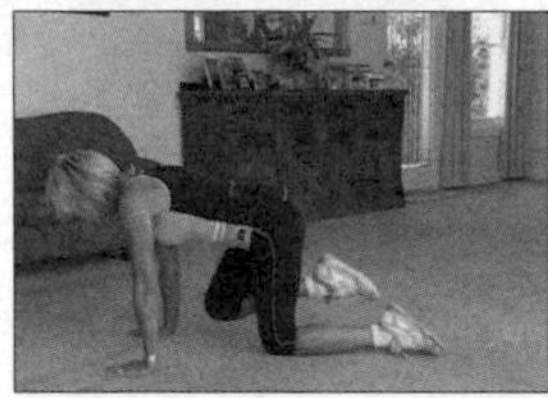
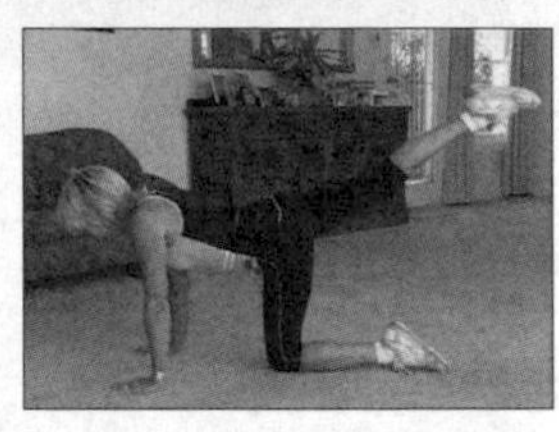

Kneel on all fours, keeping your back straight. Bring your right knee slightly forward and then extend the right leg straight back. Repeat with the left leg.

## > Arms

### *Biceps*

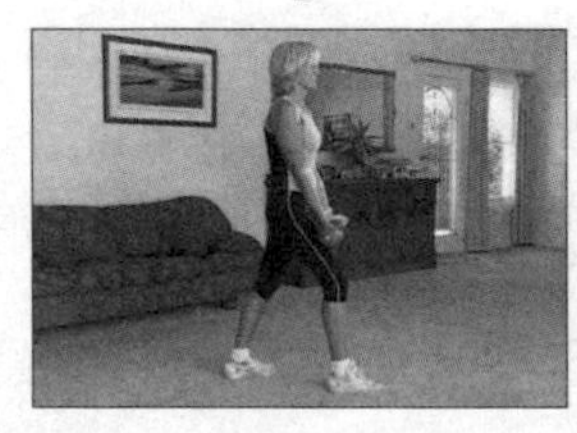
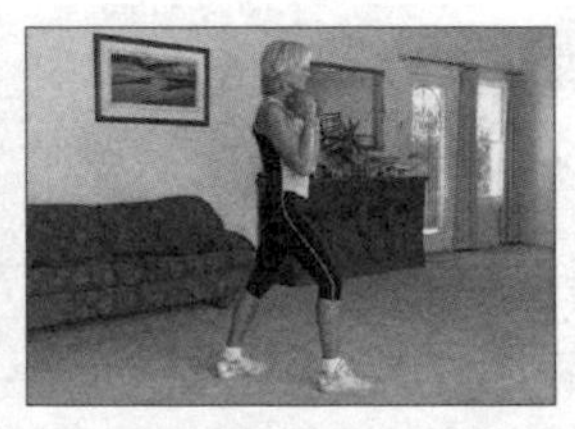

Stand with your right foot slightly ahead of the left foot, keeping your back straight. Hold the dumb-bell in your right hand, (palm facing upward), keeping the right elbow in towards the body. Slowly curl the dumb-bell forward and up towards the shoulder, then lower. After the required repetitions, repeat on the other side.

## *Triceps*

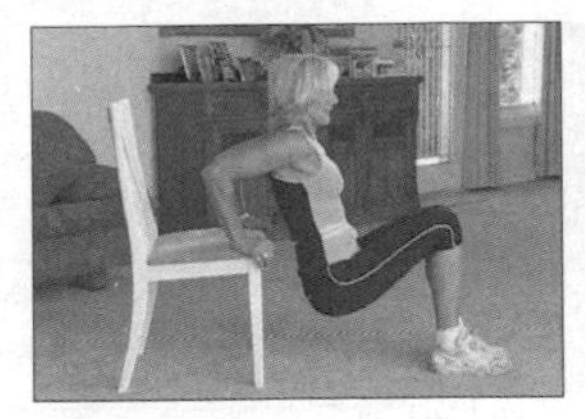

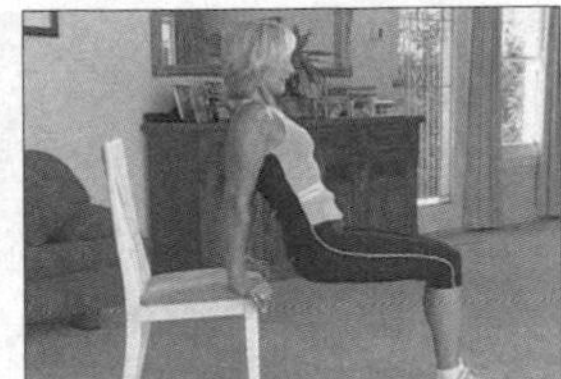

Sit on a chair. Curl your fingers on the edge of the seat with your knees bent at 90 degrees and your feet flat. Slide your bottom off the edge and keep it close to the seat. Point elbows back and in, and lower and lift yourself keeping your back straight. Beginner dips are done with knees bent. Later on, dips can be performed with legs straight.

## *Shoulders*

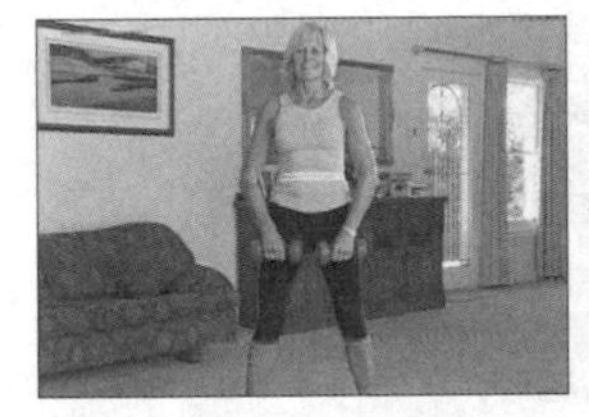

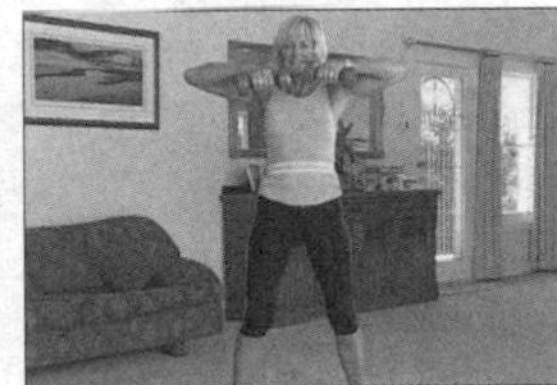

Stand with your feet shoulder-width apart, keeping your back straight. Hold the dumb bells with your palms facing your body and your arms hanging comfortably in front. Bring the weights up in a straight line to your chin, with elbows bending out and forearms finishing up parallel with the floor. Slowly lower the weights back to the starting position.

## > Tummy

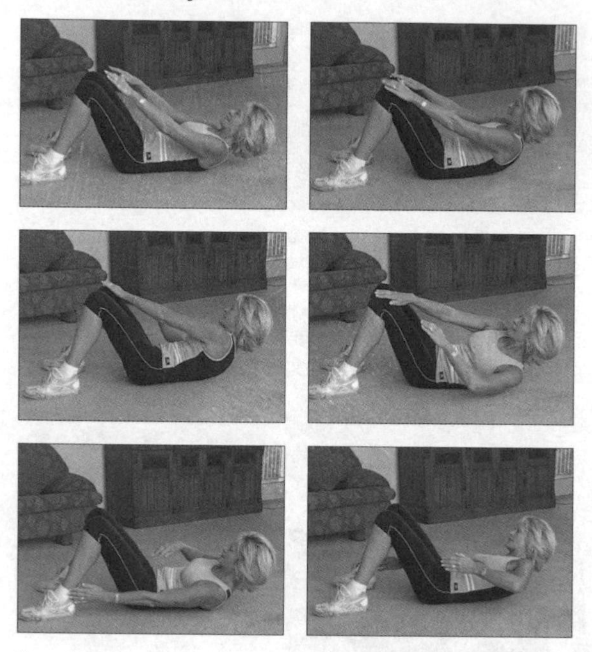

For all three crunches, lie on your back with legs bent and feet apart.

a. Slide hands towards knees, lifting head and shoulders slightly off the floor, but keeping the lower back firmly on the floor. Slowly return to starting position.

b. Reach right hand across to left knee and then left hand across to right knee before returning to starting position.

c. Reach with the right hand to the outside of the right ankle and then with the left hand to the outside of the left ankle, before lowering head and shoulders and returning to starting position.

Please always keep your lower back firmly on the floor.

## > Boobs

### *Flies*

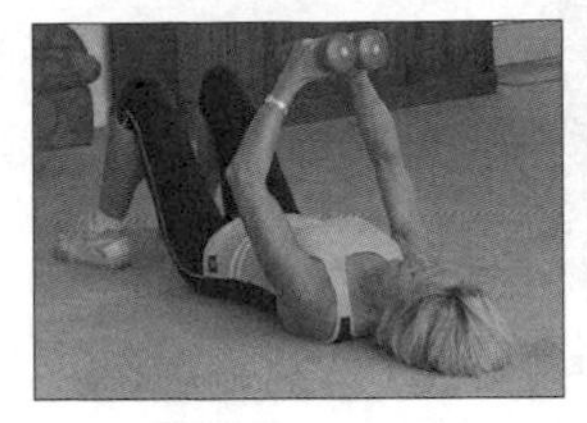
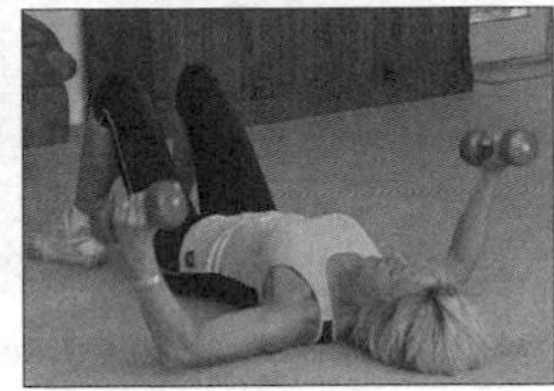

Lie on your back, legs bent, feet slightly apart. Hold the dumb-bells with arms straight up above your chest (palms facing each other). Gently lower the arms out and down until the upper arms are on the floor, elbows bent, hands up. Return the dumb-bells slowly to the starting position.

### *Push-up* A

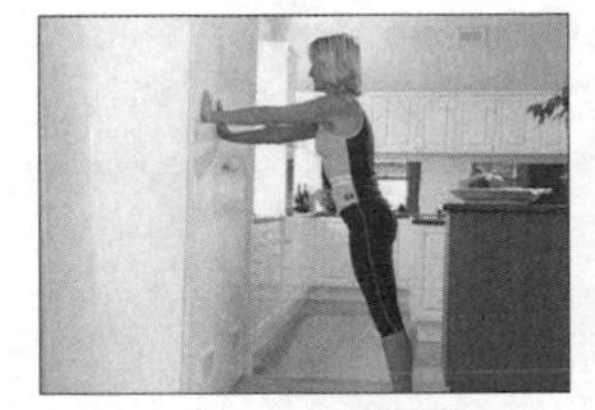
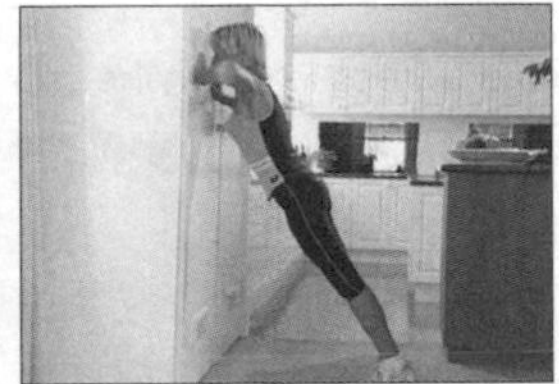

Stand (with your feet flat and almost together) facing the wall about 2.5-3 shoe lengths away. Place hands flat on the wall, shoulder width apart. Keeping the body and legs in a straight line, bend your arms at the elbows and lower yourself towards the wall. Gently push back to the starting position.

### *Push-up* B

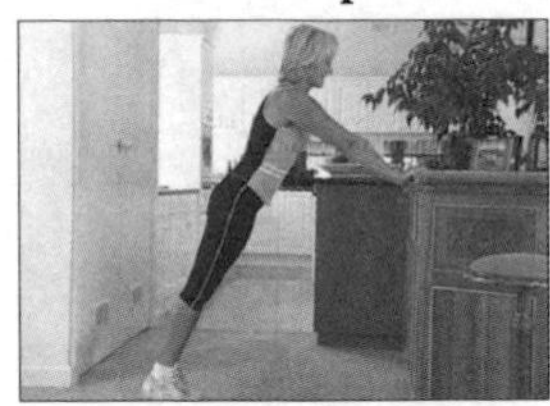
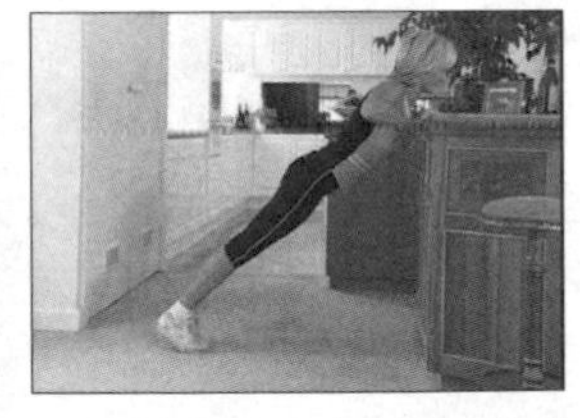

As in Push-up A, but using a waist high bench instead of the wall.

## *Push-up* C

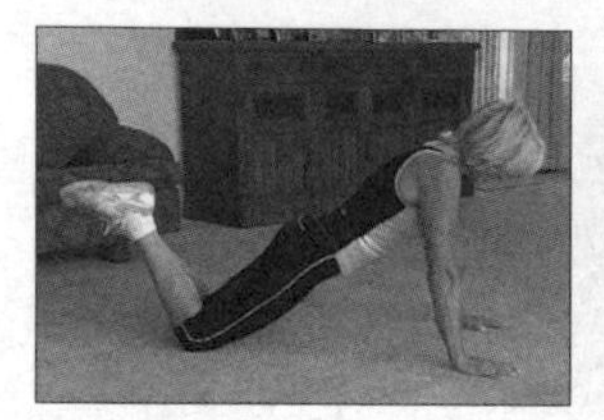
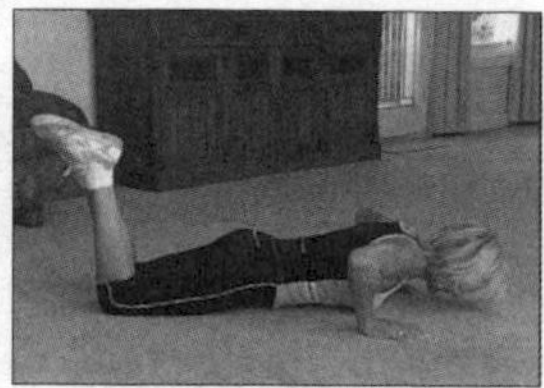

Kneel on all fours, hands shoulder-width apart, knees almost together. 'Walk' hands forward and lift lower legs, until a straight line is formed from head to knees. Hands should be directly below shoulders. Bend elbows and gently lower towards the floor maintaining the straight position from head to knees. Push up, straightening arms.

Note for men only:
These Boob exercises are for Brilliant pecs, Big pecs, Beautiful pecs. Call them whatever you want.

And men, if you wish, you can progress to doing the push-ups off your feet rather than your knees.

# OUMs - other useful movements

Do some OUMs before or after your walk, and include some neck and back movements regularly, especially if you have an office job or drive a car for long periods of time.

My daughters, Anna and Amanda, are both highly qualified Physiotherapists and have given us a list of OUMs.

Let's move down the body, from head to foot and do a few useful movements.

You can do these any time but it's best to do them before you do your **SBW** strength business.

Just do the **OUMs** ***once*** in each session.

Some of the OUMs are **L**imbering movements or warm-ups and the other are **H**olds i.e. you hold in one position for around ten seconds. We'll call them **L** Movements and **H** Movements.

OUMs relate to the following body bits.

Neck

Shoulders

Chest

Sides

Back

Hamstrings

Thighs/Quads

Calves

Feet

**L** Neck

**L** Shoulders

**H** Chest

**L** Sides

**L** Back

**H** Hamstrings

**H** Thighs/Quads

**H** Calves

**L** Feet

## > OUM Exercises

*Follow the pictures as Sue describes how to do the exercises.*

### *Neck*

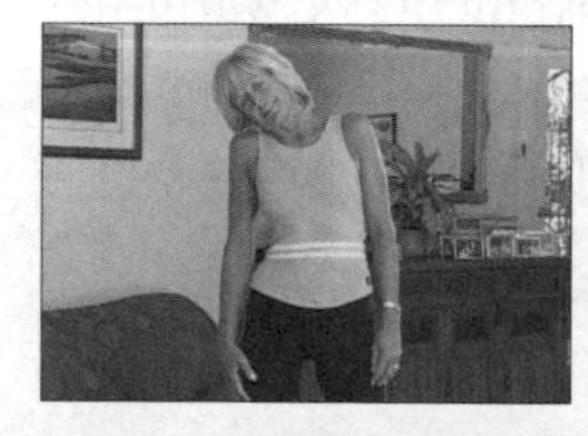
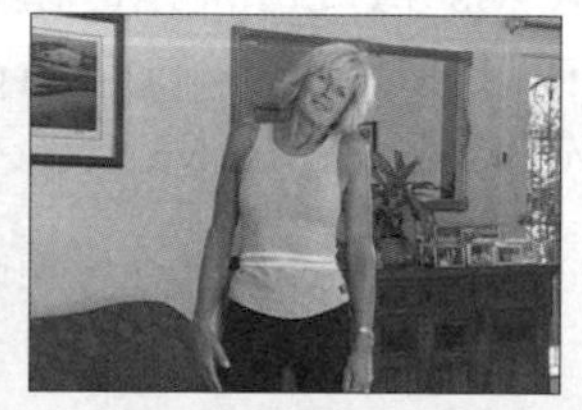
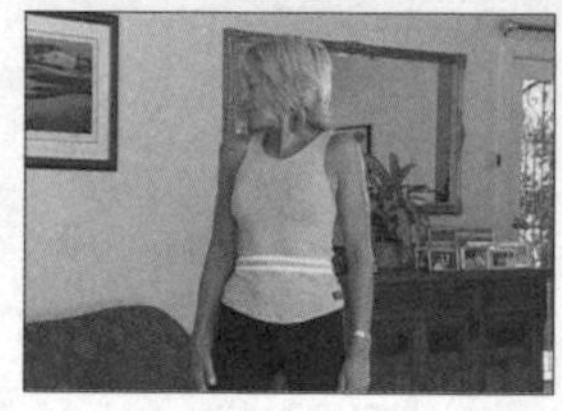
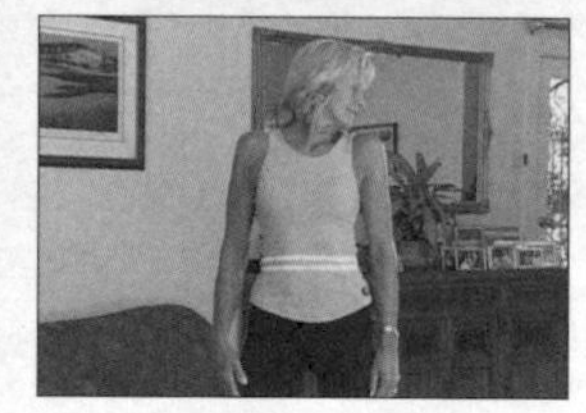

Stand with feet apart, arms by side. Tilt head slowly to one side (left ear towards left shoulder), then slowly to the other side (right ear towards right shoulder). Return head to straight position. Repeat three times. Rotate head to look beyond left shoulder, then slowly rotate the other side to look beyond right shoulder. Repeat three times.

Gently does it - don't do jerky movements, and do not do circles.

## *Shoulders*

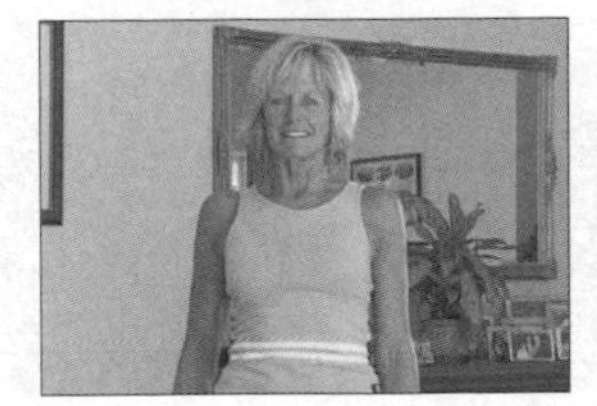
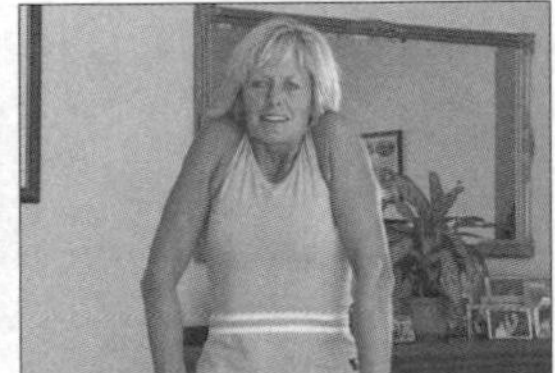

Stand with feet apart, arms by side keeping arms down, hunch shoulders slightly forward, roll them gently upward and then pull shoulders back firmly before relaxing them down to the starting position. Repeat three times.

## *Chest*

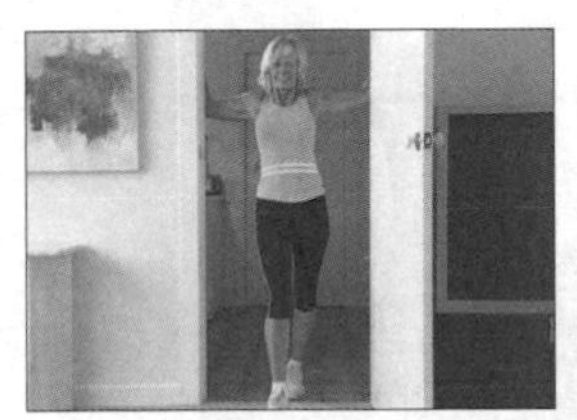
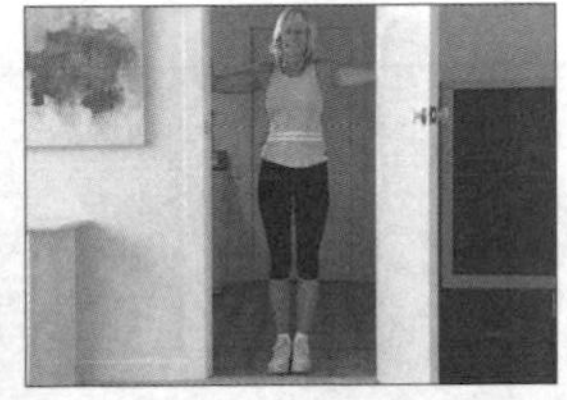
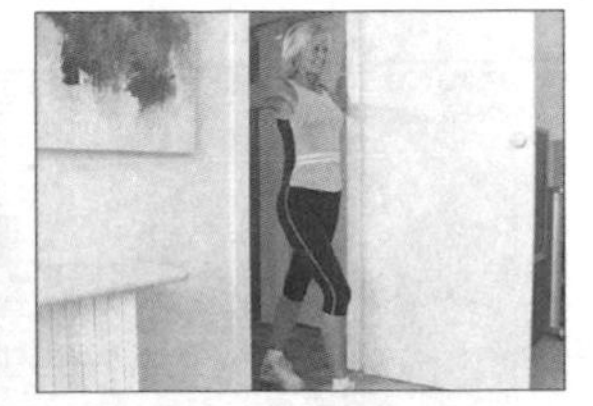

Stand in a doorway, body straight, feet almost together. Bend your arms at the elbows and raise your arms so that the upper arms are parallel with the floor and your palms are flat against the door frame. Step slowly forward with one leg until the shoulders are back and a chest stretch can be felt. Hold this position for ten seconds.

## *Sides*

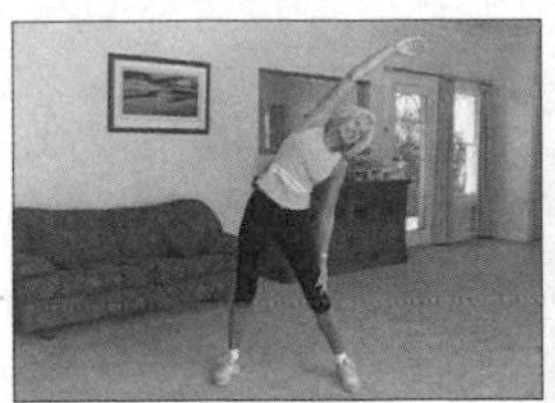
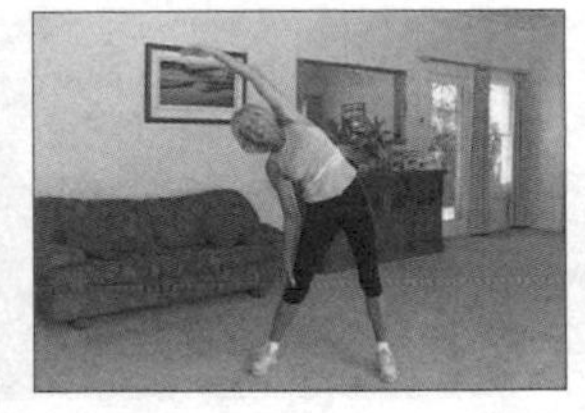
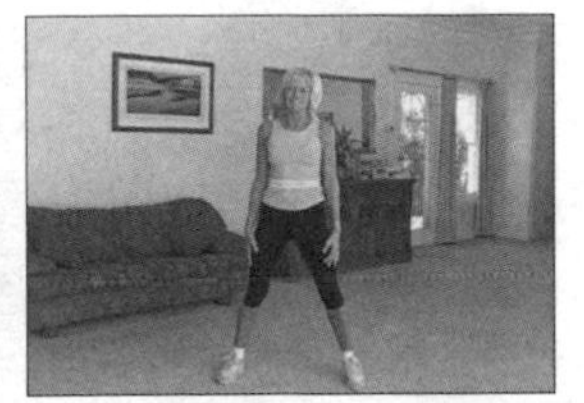

Stand with feet shoulder width apart, arms relaxed by side. Lift the right arm slowly out and up from your side, keeping it relaxed but almost straight. Slide the left arm down the left leg, gently reaching high above the head with the right arm. Slowly bring the arm back to your side. Repeat to the other side. Repeat both right and left three times.

## *Back*

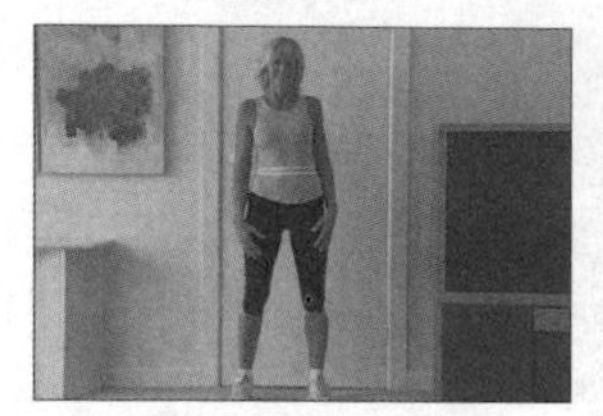
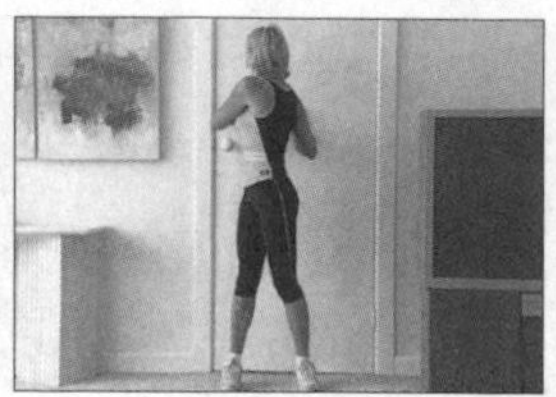
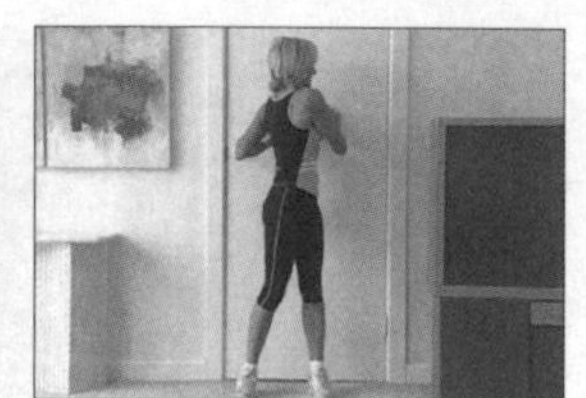

Stand with your back to the wall, feet flat and apart, about a shoe length away from the wall. Slowly turn right towards the wall with both hands reaching towards it. Gently turn the upper body back and reach left towards the wall behind you. Repeat three times.

## *Hamstrings*

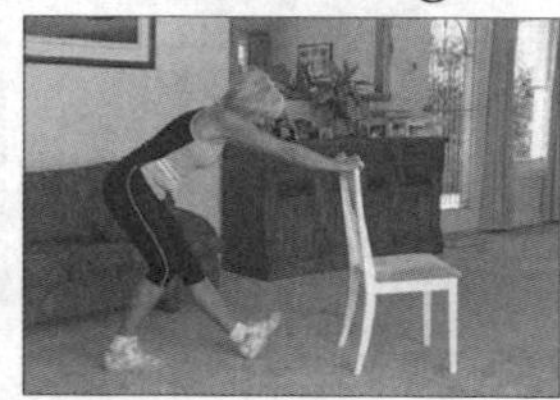
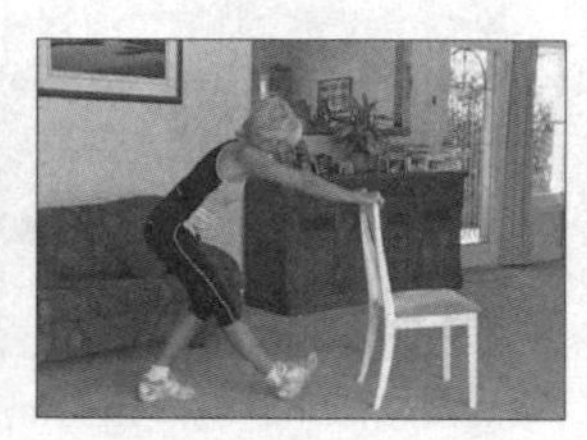

Stand behind a chair, holding the top with both hands. Place one foot well in front of the other. Slowly bend the back leg at the knee and press back into a 'sitting' position, while pointing the toes of the front straight leg up. Hold for ten seconds, then repeat with the other leg forward.

## *Thighs / Quads*

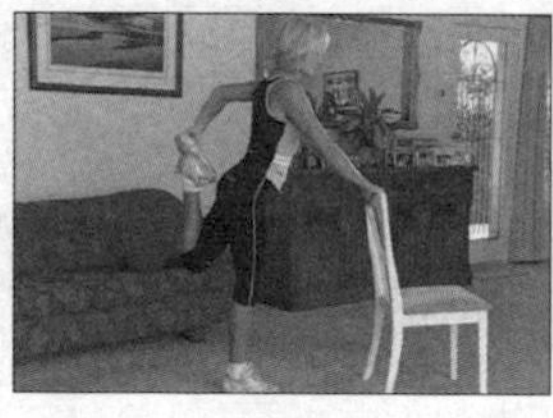
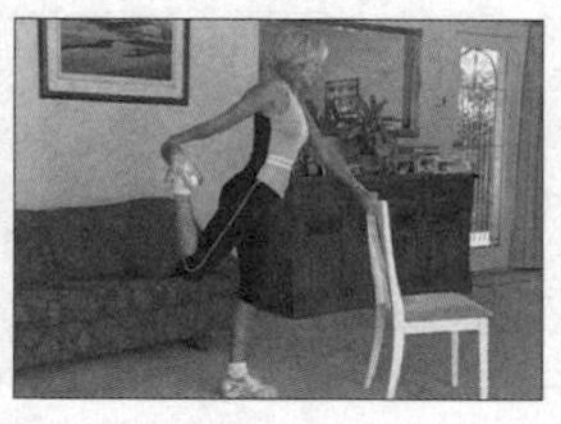

Stand up straight behind a chair, holding onto the top with the right hand. Bend the left leg back at the knee, and hold onto the foot with the left hand. Gently pull the bent leg back until the stretch is felt. Hold for ten seconds, then repeat with the other side.

## Calves

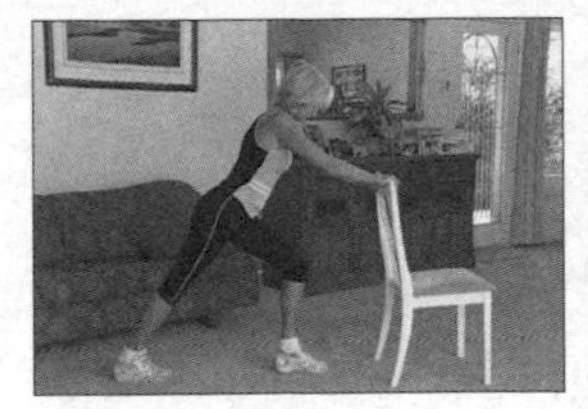
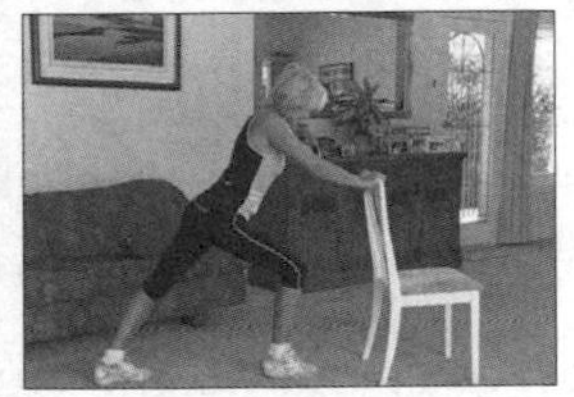

Stand behind the chair, holding onto the top with both hands. Place one foot well in front of the other, with feet in line. Bend the front leg while keeping the back leg straight with the heel on the floor. Gently press forward until the stretch is felt in the calf muscle of the back leg. Hold for ten seconds, then repeat with the other leg forward.

## Feet

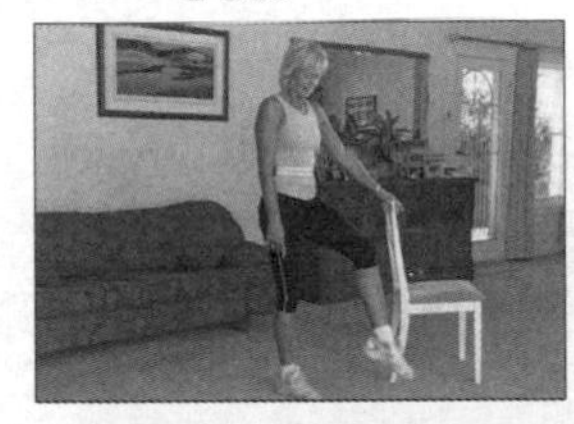
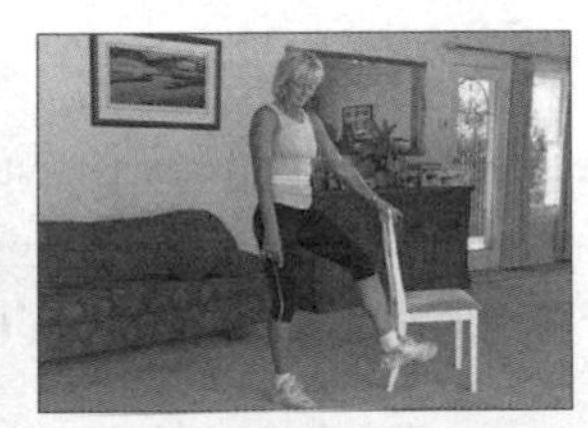
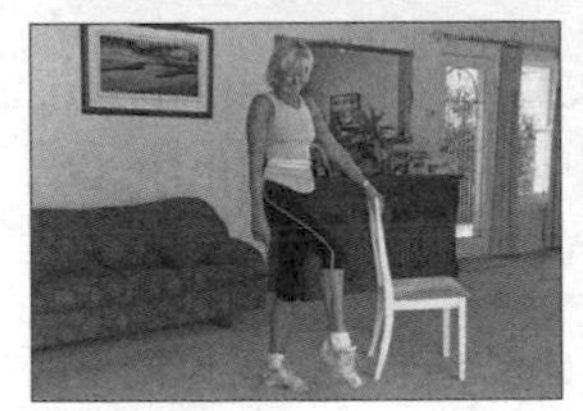
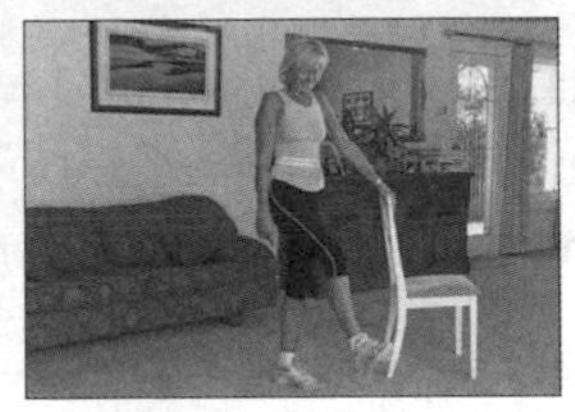

Hold onto the chair. Stand on one leg and slowly circle the other foot five times in one direction, and then five times in the opposite direction. Repeat with the other leg.

# How are you travelling?

No excuse if you are travelling. Check into a hotel by a park or a beach. A swimming pool is also very handy.

Use your briefcase as a hand-weight or unpack half your clothes and use that bag as a hand-weight instead of a dumb-bell.

Push-ups, triceps work using a chair and abdominal tightening are easy – you don't need a gym for this. Hotel fire escapes are great. If there's a fire you go down the stairs, and when there's no fire you go up the stairs.

What I do is this.

First, check that the fire escape door will open from the inside and outside, so you can get back in. I go down a few flights of stairs then I walk up the stairs. **(Don't do this if you're not fit.)**

Then I catch the elevator down and walk up the stairs again. I keep doing this until I've had enough – but not until I'm exhausted. (The hotel maids think I'm crazy!)

Personally, I don't keep walking *down* the stairs as it bothers my back, but you can walk down as well if you wish.

Activity

# Coping >

Eating

## > COPING IS THE C IN A C E <

We need to get one thing straight and not too many health gurus and diet gurus realise this.

You are not **under stress** – stress is inside you. Stress is on the inside and PRESSURE is on the outside.

So you are under **pressure** and this causes a **stress response**, which can be positive, negative or neutral.

The human body loves positive stress responses – there is no downside here at all. The human body does not enjoy negative stress responses piled one on top of the other because this causes the body to break down and become unwell.

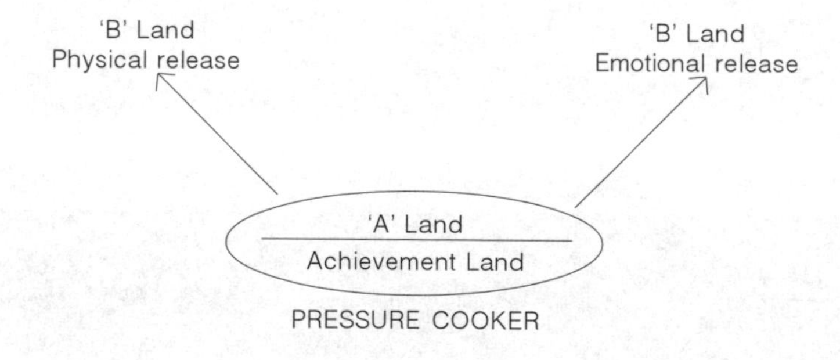


We all like achieving – it makes us feel good. To achieve something, we need to have some pressure applied and this causes a response.

If you have absolutely no pressure, this is sort of like 'zombie land'. Retirement can be a bit like that. Retired people have to be *really* careful that they don't go down-hill fast. Retirement is a funny word.

If you are already tired, why do you want to get re-tired?

Where people go wrong is this – they forget that to be really good *in* the pressure cooker of life, you need to get *out* of it on a regular basis.

This escape mechanism can be either physical or emotional.

I have discussed with many people what they consider the best ways to get out of the pressure cooker and re-vitalise or re-energise their minds and their bodies.

Here is a Relaxation List (by no means complete). Choose several and place them in your life regularly. To score your Living*life* points, you need to do one or two each day.

## > Relaxation List

- Go to one of these destinations – a mountain, forest, beach, stream or pool – sit there, walk there or lie there
- Watch a sunset
- Watch a sunrise
- Go to a movie
- Have coffee with a friend
- Sit in the sunshine
- Lie in the sunshine
- Sip a glass of really good wine
- Read a book
- Jump in the ocean
- Have a warm bath
- Light a candle

- Listen to relaxing music
- Do some deep breathing
- Have a massage
- Have a facial
- Plan your next three-day break
- Have a cup of tea and do a crossword puzzle
- Close your eyes and dream of good things
- Call someone you haven't seen for a while
- Go to an old-folks home and have a chat
- Learn Tai Chi

> When you have a problem, there may be more than one way to tackle it.

Think of the alternative approaches and if things are not clear, involve somebody else and seek their advice.

Women are usually good at seeking comfort and help from others.

Men are usually not so good at this. We need to get better.

> An attitude boost is most helpful. Remember Tom Cruise in the movie *Cocktail*? He always had a motivational book under the bar. Positive re-inforcement on a regular basis is excellent.

> Check out your behaviour type – A, B, C or maybe AB. Work on it if you need to. Be aware of your responses to people and events.

Monitor your aggression levels and how things build up inside you – and how long it takes you to calm down.

- Think good things and dream a little.
- Do you have your next three-day spouse break or partner break planned? Well, do it. Ring the travel shop and get some brochures.

**> Did you get your laugh, hug, relaxation, sleep and good person points today? <**

If yes – sensational. If no – how come?

***The Great Australian Diet*** is very keen on good **Coping** skills as well as good **Activity** and **Eating** skills.

Why?

Because if you are doing the things we are talking about here, it makes you feel so much better about yourself and about life.

Go to your weekly 91 DAY SUCCESS CHART and aim at scoring the maximum number of coping points as you travel through the program.

It certainly makes a difference.

# Today's 91 Day coping list

Every day you need to ask yourself these questions –

| | | |
|---|---|---|
| Good sleep last night? | Yes | ☐ |
| Deep breathing? | Yes | ☐ |
| Laugh? | Yes | ☐ |
| Hug? | Yes | ☐ |
| Something good for someone else? | Yes | ☐ |
| Another 'thing' from the Relaxation List? | Yes | ☐ |

Activity

Coping

Eating >

## > EATING IS THE E IN A C E <

Eating is easy.

Do the right thing.

Get smart.

Your 'machine' is depending on you.

Follow the guidelines.

And smile.

# The four keys

> BASIC AND BONUS
>
> TWO-THIRDS, ONE-THIRD
>
> RULE OF 15
>
> H.I. INDEX

## > BASIC AND BONUS

There are two food groups in the world.

- BASIC Foods are Plant.
- BONUS Foods are Not Plant.

Fish is the best Bonus Food.

Plant Foods are vegetables, fruits, nuts, grains and seeds.

How do I know that Basic Food or Plant Food is Basic?

As the Poms would say, *'It's bleedin' obvious'*.

Basically, the human machine **can live a long and healthy life on Plant Food alone.**

The human machine **cannot live a long and healthy life on just flesh food and food of animal origin**, although one could be forgiven for thinking (if you read the latest bunch of diet experts) that the opposite is true. If sceptics want to get aggressive on this one – then go and research a little harder.

The evidence is loud and clear.

You see, Plant Foods have thousands of micro-nutrients which together make the machine run superbly. Bonus Foods have far fewer nutrients. It is also strange that Plant Foods are mainly **carbohydrates** with some protein and a few plants also contain some fat.

Now there's a revelation!

## > TWO-THIRDS, ONE-THIRD

The best rule of nutrition ever invented is this – and I invented it.

At least two-thirds of the food that goes into your mouth **must** be of plant origin.

That's what the longest living races of people in the world seem to do.

It makes perfect sense.

Go back to the East versus West section and have a look at the food intake charts.

I didn't need to make this up or invent it – these are merely the facts of life – **Real Life**.

## > RULE OF 15

This rule is another cornerstone of the *The Great Australian Diet*. It is the rule that causes the biggest shift in ATTITUDE and underpins the SUCCESS of my program.

Eat small amounts of at least **15 Plant Foods each day**.

My experience tells me that the Rule of 15 has an extremely positive influence on –

- Weight control
- Energy levels, and
- Cancer risk

How do you achieve the **Rule of 15?**

You eat/nibble different varieties, different colours, small portions of vegetables, fruits, nuts, grains and seeds.

Impossible? Not so.

Here's a list of the foods and liquids I ate and drank yesterday. (in no particular order) This shows you how you can achieve the all important variety of foods –

- banana
- carrot
- strawberries
- coffee
- brussels sprouts
- passionfruit
- grapes
- lamb chop
- spring onions
- mandarin
- corn
- raspberries
- water
- soy and linseed bread
- small can of sardines
- yoghurt
- olives
- soy milk
- alfalfa
- avocado
- almonds
- prunes
- tomato
- beetroot
- soybeans
- red wine

So 19 of these are Plant Foods (20 with red wine!).

Remember you can't count refined or processed foods.

**Refined products don't count**! White bread doesn't count. Table sugar doesn't count. Coco Pops don't count.

Why not?

If you can't tell me why not by now, read on ...

Total 26 different foods and drinks – most of them plant.

You don't need to eat all of these, but after a few days, you begin to broaden your horizons.

As well as these foods, there are others that you may wish to consider.

I must be nuts you say?

Not so – it has become a habit to eat little bits and pieces of whatever I can find. I repeat, VARIETY is the name of the game.

For breakfast at home, I would usually have six or seven different fruits – not seven whole pieces of fruit. In the fridge, there is always a bowl of chopped fruit and the bowl contains such fruits as nectarines, plums, apricots, grapes, apple, passionfruit, blueberries etc.

Then I often follow up with grilled tomato on toast to which I add a teaspoon of olive oil – great! (No butter, no spreads.)

Lunch – I go down to the salad bar and have six or seven different things on my soy and linseed bread sandwich.

Dinner – Fish or meat and two vegetables. No way, I have six vegetables! It's no more trouble.

Also, there is no such thing as a 'serving' in *The Great Australian Diet.*

A few grapes count as 'one' Plant Food. A bite of banana counts as 'one' Plant Food. Three or four olives count as 'one'. A half slice of soy and linseed bread counts as 'one'. You don't need large quantities of food – you just don't.

## > H.I. INDEX

Humans have a habit of messing around with food.

This used to be uncommon – now it's *very* common.

Not good. Not good at all.

So H.I. is the level of Human Interference, or in other words how much or how badly humans have changed the food from natural to not-so-natural.

Get it?

Good.

*The Great Australian Diet* steers you away from high H.I. foods, especially anything that is processed or deep fried.

This is so important, we'll do an H.I. briefing in the next couple of chapters.

Complicated? No way. It's fun working out all the ways that humans can stuff up good food.

# Think and win

Why would I call this chapter 'Think and win'?

I'll tell you why.

Because unless your lottery numbers come up, winners in life generally need to use a little brain power.

... just a little.

As I've said, this is not rocket science and you don't need to count grams or carbs or calories or refer to scales or a complicated index.

In fact it is so easy, you're going to get the hang of it really quickly.

I'm going to give you the guidelines, along with some examples – then you'll be able to work out the H.I. of anything!

Here we go ...

## > H.I. Guidelines

H.I. is all about humans interfering with our food.

What do I mean by interfered with? Well, let's go through some of the ways that foods are messed up.

Before we start this list, let's give nature some credit for creating decent, wholesome food.

So we'll begin with an H.I. Index of 0 (or zero), for a real whole food.

Then I mentally go through a list of what might have happened to a food before it was picked or killed and add an H.I. point for each of these not-so-good things.

The second stage is to work out what has happened or is happening to the food after it is 'harvested'.

The last thing you do is decide whether or not you're going to eat it, or even consume part of it!

Put simply, we add an H.I. point every time a food is interfered with.

There is only one exception here – that's when something is **deep fried**. For deep frying, we're not going to add a point to the total, we're going to **multiply the total H.I. by 2** ... i.e. we're going to double the H.I.

That's what I think about that level of interference!

Don't forget there are good oils and there are not-so-good oils. Good oils include olive oil, flaxseed and canola. We give them an **H.I. of zero** unless they have been turned into solid fat. Then they become **H.I.** 1

That's it.

Pretty simple.

Where to now?

Well the lower the H.I. of a food the better, and it is possible to have an H.I of zero, eg. water or tea without milk or sugar, regular vegetables and fruits, some fish and some meat, (kangaroo for example).

There is probably no upper limit on H.I. because there are any number of ways humans have invented to modify the food we eat (and that's being kind).

That's the beauty of *The Great Australian Diet*. You're not asked to count calories, measure servings or look up a G.I. chart.

I don't tell you not to eat this or not to eat that because you can eat anything you want to. But what will happen is that you start to wonder why you need a huge muffin instead of a third of it, three donuts instead of one or none, or two helpings of ice cream instead of one scoop on some fresh fruit. You see, all you are doing is feeding your tongue!

*The Great Australian Diet* approach is simple.

This is the way I handle it ...

I look at foods individually and then look at the whole meal.

I assess the food and the meal like this ...

Are the foods BASIC or BONUS?

Easy – plant or not plant.

Is at least two-thirds of the meal BASIC Food?

Easy – fish and salad or vegetables plus some fries. The salad and vegetables are Basic, the fish is Bonus but great Bonus because of its low H.I. The fries are 'officially' plant, but they have been totally wrecked by H.I., so I might eat three fries instead of 300!

And the last thing – is this meal helping me towards my 15 Plant Foods for the day?

The only tough decision is this ...

Can you walk away from 297 fries???

I can.

I just visualise what they would do to the inside of my human machine (not worth the risk)!

But if you want to go for it just **now** and **then** – good luck to you.

Hey – just don't do it in your **Switch On** weeks, OK?

# The H.I. list

## > Pre-'harvesting' H.I. Index – add 1

- Chemical 'enhancement'
  eg. steroids, antibiotics, fertilisers, pesticides
- Artificial growth factors
  eg. light, heat, un-natural feed
- Genetic modification

## > Post-'harvesting' H.I. Index – add 1

- Refining
- Processing
- Preservatives
- Colourings
- Additives/additions
- Subtractions
- Packaging
  eg. packet, can, bottle, box, jar, carton, tub
  (frozen is OK – H.I. zero)
- Long-term storage
- Peeled, sliced, diced, mashed, smashed, pureed
- Salting (pepper is OK)
- Sugaring
- Oiling
- Cooking
- Saucing

# Exceptions and quirkies

## > Packaging

- I don't add **H.I.** 1 for frozen food – zero is fine
- Oiling
- I don't add **H.I.** 1 for a little added
  - olive oil
  - canola oil
  - flaxseed oil
  - soy bean oil

  Zero is fine for small amounts. But if oils are **solid** eg. canola in a tub – I then add **H.I.** 1

## > Cooking

- I don't add **H.I.** 1 for
  - lightly steaming
  - lightly cooking in a wok
  - a quick drop into boiling water

  Zero is fine by me.

My cooking H.I. ratings go like this:

| | |
|---|---|
| • Lightly steaming | 0 |
| • Wok – lightly cooking | 0 |
| • Quick drop into boiling water | 0 |
| • Microwave zap | 0/1 |

I don't add **H.I.** 1 point for a microwave zap, but you might – it's your call.

| | |
|---|---|
| • Grilling | 1 |
| • Boiling | 1 |
| • Baking | 1 |
| • Roasting | 1 |
| • Smoking | 1 |
| • BBQ'ing | 2 |

But **DEEP FRYING – multiply x 2 – double** the H.I. Index.

## > Fluids

- Water is zero
- Green tea and black tea are zero

I don't add **H.I.** 1 for up to two cups of coffee per day.

I don't add **H.I.** 1 for

- Sips of skim milk
- Soy milk. Soy milk (non-G.M.) is zero

## > Sauces / Dressings

I add **H.I.** 1 for any sauce or dressing except

- (a little) olive oil and vinegar is a zero

Now check out the examples and learn the ropes ...

Here are some real life examples –

## > Example 1

***An Apple***

Might have been sprayed so wash it.

Hope it got ripe in the sunshine.

At this stage, the apple's H.I. Index is around zero.

Going along the good to not-so-good scale, the progression would be –

1 apple picked, washed and eaten whole – **H.I. still** zero

2 Grandma's apple pie (with big chunks of apple and a little pastry), apple peeled and stewed (1), sugar added (1), pastry with refined flour (1) – **H.I.** 3

3 apple muffin with a few bits of cooked apple (1), along with huge amounts of sugar (1), refined flour (1), full of fat – trans fats (1) – **H.I.** 4 or more

4 fast food apple pie, say peeled, smashed, sugar, refined flour – so I'll give it a **H.I.** 4 and then I'll double it because it's probably fried.That makes the **H.I.** 8 !

Get the idea?

After a while, you can assess a food in a few seconds ... good, fair, maybe a bite or two, disaster.

## > Example 2

***Take a Potato***

Let's pretend it grew up OK – H.I. zero

What did I do to it?

– sliced, diced, peeled or mashed – there's a **1**

What did I add to it?

– salt and butter – add **2 more H.I.s**

How did I cook it?

– baked with olive oil – add **1**

That's a total H.I. of 4

If I were rating fries, the H.I. is immediately doubled because of the deep frying, so I'd give it a H.I. of at least 6 (wouldn't you?)

And don't forget it's a QUANTITY thing as well. A couple of small, real potatoes versus a truck-full of fries.

Remember, we're not trying to get too technical here. This is not an exam. It's a great way of working out how junky or useless the food is, or on the other hand, how real it is. Most importantly, you must begin to recognise the factors that give foods a high H.I. and start to avoid them.

## Example 3

***Chicken***

Here are some chicken ideas for you …

How was it raised?

– under lights – H.I. 1

What did it eat?

– un-natural pellets – H.I. 1

Other elements

– given steroids and antibiotics – H.I. 1 and **add another 1**

What happened to it?

– killed, plucked and packed in plastic or foam – H.I. 1

What part of it am I eating?

– breast – H.I. zero

– legs and skin – H.I. 1 for each

How was it cooked?

– boiled – H.I. 1

– grilled – H.I. 1

– deep fried – multiply H.I. by 2

Has it been re-heated? H.I. 1

Let's say we are eating re-heated chicken leg with the skin which had been deep fried, we bought it from a supermarket wrapped in foam and plastic and it had originally been force-fed pellets under lights and given steroids to make it grow quicker.

I'd give it about a 13 !

In fact it should have flashing red lights all around it.

Are you getting the picture? Whether you think its H.I. is 10, 12, 14 or 200, doesn't really matter. What does matter is that this re-heated chicken is a disaster.

I'd rather have a glass of red wine or starve!

## > Example 4

***Fish***

What sort of fish?

– deep sea, cold water fish – **H.I.** zero

– farm grown fish – **H.I.** 1

– bottom dwelling crustaceans – **H.I.** 1

How did it arrive?

– straight from market – **H.I.** zero

– in a can – **H.I.** zero **or H.I.** 1 – it's your call

How was it cooked?

– wok with canola oil or lightly steamed – **H.I.** zero

– wok with saturated oil – **H.I.** 1

– grilled or baked – I'd say a **1** but you may call it a **zero**

– deep fried – multiply **H.I. by 2**

Was anything added?

– salt – **H.I.** 1

– sauces – **H.I.** 1

– lemon – **H.I.** zero

The fish we have prepared was a deep sea fish (salmon) which came straight from the market, was cooked in a wok with canola oil and with some added lemon, chives or parsley.

Hey the H.I. is close to zero. You beauty! Add a few vegetables and you're really rocking and rolling.

Get the picture?

This is simple – and this is fun.

It's your call now because you have all the basic information at your fingertips.

As I said – all you need to do is to **Think and win**.

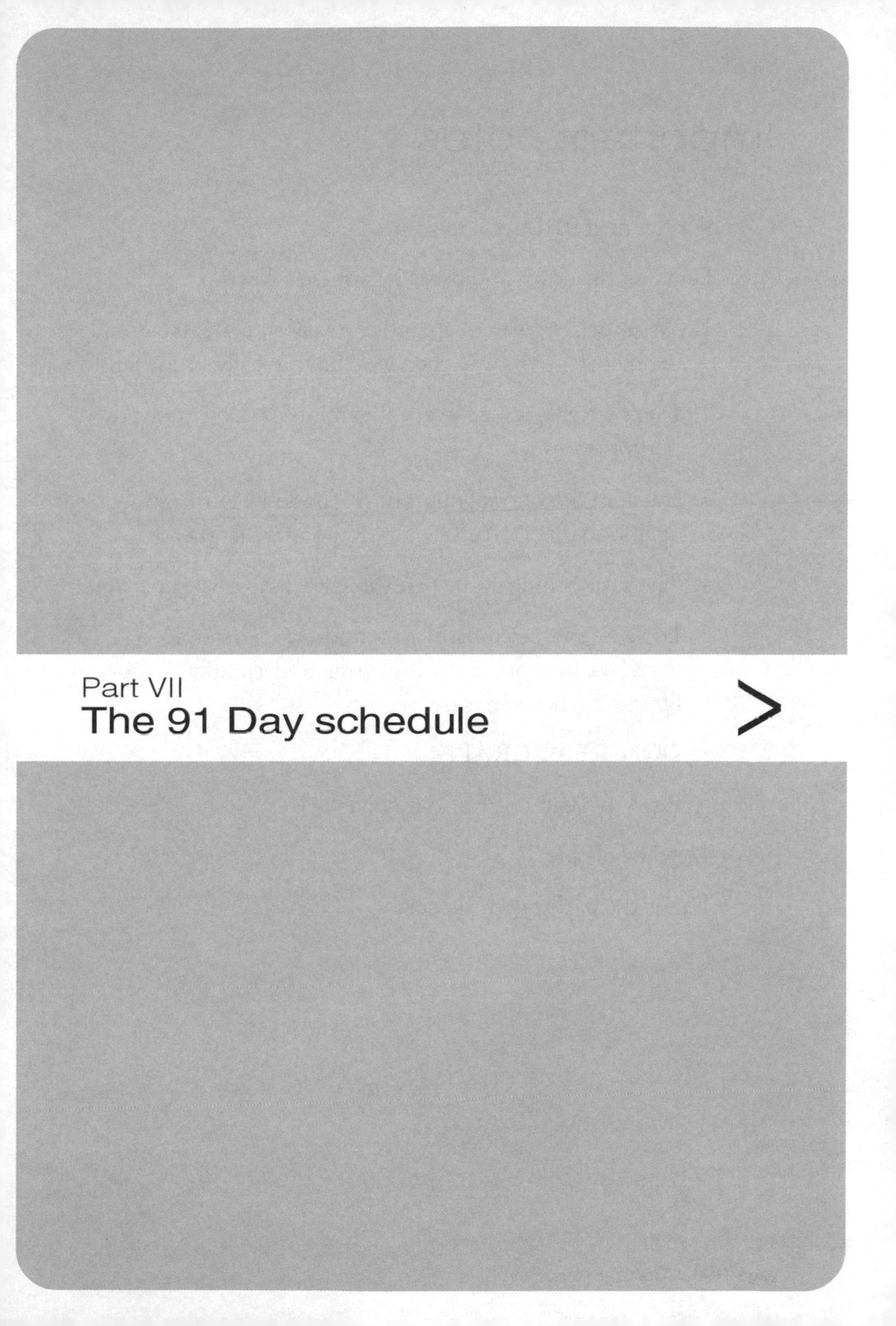

Part VII

# The 91 Day schedule

# Important notes

For the next 91 Days, I'm your coach.

Don't let me down and don't let yourself down.

1. We ***must*** get away to a good start. We'll plateau a couple of times along the way, then we'll have a really strong finish.
2. ***Don't*** weigh yourself every five minutes. Do it now, then not for two weeks.
3. You ***must*** do your walking – brisk if possible. Put the walking appointments IN YOUR DIARY, one week ahead.
4. The eating thing in the first three weeks is ***very important.***
5. Look at the pictures of Sue and do the simple B.A.T. exercises for your bottoms, arms and tummy – they're fantastic (the exercises).
6. **DON'T EAT CRAP!**
7. Read through the Fail-Safe Snacks.

They're fail-safe.

This is the pathway to success.

# More important notes

At the beginning of each week, there is a **Success Chart**.

Don't freak out when you see it. Just browse through for a start and then each day, pop in the numbers.

For example each day you score –

- 2 points **each** for walking and Rule of 15, and
- 1 point **each** for B.A.T. and OUM exercises, Two-thirds, One-Third rule, breakfast and each 'thing' from the Relaxation List.

It's really easy and IT WORKS.

At the end of each week, transfer your total to the Scoreboard on the inside **back** cover of the book.

ACCOUNTABILITY is the name of the game. It is **you** looking after **you** – the greatest machine on earth.

Should I wish you Good Luck?

No, because it's got nothing to do with luck.

Just do it!

# Dr John Tickell's 91 Day Success Chart

*At the completion of each week, transfer your weekly Livinglife points to the Scoreboard on the inside back cover*

| ACE | Week 1 | M | T | W | T | F | S | S | Living*life* Points My Total | Goal | Max |
|---|---|---|---|---|---|---|---|---|---|---|---|
| A1 | Did I do my walk today? 2 points per day – Goal: 14 points per week. *If you walk minimum of 5 days per week – score 4 bonus points* | | | | | | | | | 14 | 14 |
| A2 | Did I do my strength work today? 1 point per day – Goal: 4 or 5 points per week | | | | | | | | | 5 | 7 |
| A3 | Did I do my OUMs today? 1 point per day – Goal: 4 or 5 points per week | | | | | | | | | 5 | 7 |
| | ACTIVITY TOTALS | | | | | | | | | 24 | 28 |
| E1 | Did I eat/nibble my 15 Plant Foods today? 2 points per day – Goal: 12 points per week | | | | | | | | | 12 | 14 |
| E2 | Did I do the 2/3, 1/3 routine today? 1 point per day – Goal: 6 points per week | | | | | | | | | 6 | 7 |
| E3 | Did I eat breakfast today? 1 point per day – Goal: 6 points per week | | | | | | | | | 6 | 7 |
| | EATING TOTALS | | | | | | | | | 24 | 28 |
| C1 | Did I have a laugh and give someone a hug today? 1 point per day – Goal: 6 points per week | | | | | | | | | 6 | 7 |
| C2 | Did I do some deep breathing and another relaxation thing today? 1 point per day – Goal: 6 points per week | | | | | | | | | 6 | 7 |
| C3 | Did I have a good sleep last night? 1 point per day – Goal: 6 points per week | | | | | | | | | 6 | 7 |
| C4 | Did I do something good for, or be nice to someone else today? 1 point per day – Goal: 6 points per week | | | | | | | | | 6 | 7 |
| | COPING TOTALS | | | | | | | | | 24 | 28 |
| | WEEKLY GRAND TOTAL | | | | | | | | | 72 | 84 |

*Switch-On weeks – aim at minimum of 60 LLPs per week*

*Switch-Off weeks – why not aim at the same number of LLPs?*

# Week 1 - Activity Schedule

Please mark these sessions in your diary - now - for this coming week.
Make the appointments with yourself.
The B.A.T and OUMs are laid out for you on Pages 143 and 150.

| | **Monday Day 1** | **Tuesday Day 2** | **Wednesday Day 3** | **Thursday Day 4** | **Friday Day 5** | **Saturday Day 6** | **Sunday Day 7** |
|---|---|---|---|---|---|---|---|
| 1% | | Walk 25 min. | | Walk 25 min. | | Walk 25 min. | Walk 25 min. |
| SBW | | BAT Exercises Sets: 1 Reps: 6 | | BAT Exercises Sets: 1 Reps: 6 | | BAT Exercises Sets: 1 Reps: 6 | BAT Exercises Sets: 1 Reps: 6 |
| Refer to the BAT exercises on page 143 | | | | | | | |
| OUMs | | OUMs … once | | OUMs … once | | OUMs … once | OUMs … once |
| Refer to the OUM exercises on page 150 | | | | | | | |

- We are moving one percent of our life i. e. 100 minutes per week.
- The strength work – SBW – these are suggested repetition levels.
- The weights you use? It depends … Try 3 kg weights for women and 5 kg for men. You need to know you are lifting something but don't overdo it. Starting out with lighter weights is just fine.
- If you get muscle soreness or strain, back right off for a couple of days or use lighter weights.

# Week 1 - Day 1

### *Breakfast*

- Glass of water
- Equivalent of one piece of fruit only e.g. half a banana, half an apple, or a few grapes, three or four prunes, etc.
- Grilled tomatoes
  pepper is O.K. – no salt
  no bread – no toast
- Cup of green tea or Jasmine tea

### *Snack*

- Glass of water
- Equivalent of half a piece of fruit – half a banana or a few grapes
- Sip of soy milk or skim milk or smoothie
- Spoon of low fat yoghurt
- Coffee or tea OK

### *Lunch*

- Glass of water
- Bowl of vegetable soup or minestrone

### *Snack*

- Glass of water
- Same as morning snack

### *Dinner*

- Glass of water
- Bowl of vegetable soup or minestrone

### *Evening Snack or Get Up During the Night Snack*

- Two spoons of low fat yoghurt
- Sip of smoothie, soy milk/skim milk
- Cup of minestrone

### *Alternative - Day 1*

As an alternative to this **Day 1** - you may choose to have vegetable soup only.
That's it ... and a spoon of low fat yoghurt here and there if you wish.

### *Notes:*

Day 1 is a **cleansing** day.

Cut up a number of fruits in a bowl and have it sitting in the fridge.

This is getting your numbers up, working on The Rule of 15.

Remember, The Rule of 15 kicks in on Day 3.

Snacks – Every diet has snacks. I am not forcing you to eat snacks.

If I'm excited or busy, I don't get hungry, but on passing the fridge, I may have two teaspoons of yoghurt or a sip of skim milk or smoothie as *hunger prevention*.

You don't need a whole glass of milk or smoothie or a whole tub of yoghurt – just a little will do.

Minestrone often includes some rice or pasta. A little whole-grain rice is OK – pasta is not. A sprinkle of cheese is OK – no meat.

Coffee – not milk coffee – with a little milk is OK.

# Week 1 - Day 1

Your body may not like you for a few days. It depends how different this eating is compared with your 'normal' eating.

**It is not unusual to feel this way if your system has been full of 'Human Interfered' with foods for a long time.**

**The cleansing of toxins from your bloodstream may take seven to 10 days and then your machine will be starting to fire.**

**If you are going to the bathroom more often (even at night), then so be it. When your waterworks are pushing out clearer fluids, that means you are winning.**

**If you need to do the hard yards, then do it. Don't wimp out on me.**

**It's all good.**

***Simple Smoothie***

2 cups soy and/or skim milk
A few spoons of low fat yoghurt
Any fruits – e.g. banana, mango, berries, peach etc.
1 teaspoon of honey (optional)
Few drops of vanilla essence.

Mix all ingredients and keep smoothie in fridge.

THIS IS FOR SIPPING, not guzzling.

## Activity

| | |
|---|---|
| A gentle walk if you wish.<br>The real routine starts on Day 2 | ☐ |

## Coping

| | | |
|---|---|---|
| Good sleep last night? | Yes | ☐ |
| Deep breathing? | Yes | ☐ |
| Laugh? | Yes | ☐ |
| Hug? | Yes | ☐ |
| Something good for someone else? | Yes | ☐ |
| Another 'thing' from the Relaxation List? | Yes | ☐ |

Fill out your Living*life* Points on your weekly Success Chart

# Week 1 - Day 2

***Breakfast***

- Glass of water
- Equivalent of one piece of fruit only e.g. half a banana, half an apple, or a few grapes, three or four prunes, etc.
- Grilled tomatoes
  pepper is O.K. – no salt
  no bread – no toast
- Cup of green tea or Jasmine tea

***Snack***

- Glass of water
- Equivalent of half a piece of fruit – half a banana or a few grapes
- Sip of soy milk or skim milk or smoothie
- Spoon of low fat yoghurt
- Coffee or tea OK

***Lunch***

- Glass of water
- Bowl of vegetable soup or minestrone

***Snack***

- Glass of water
- Same as morning snack

***Dinner***

- Glass of water
- Bowl of vegetable soup or minestrone

***Evening Snack or Get Up During the Night Snack***

- Two spoons of low fat yoghurt
- Sip of smoothie, soy milk/skim milk
- Cup of minestrone

***Alternative - Day 2***

As an alternative to this **Day 2** - you may choose to have vegetable soup only.
That's it ... and a spoon of low fat yoghurt here and there if you wish.

***Notes:***

Day 2 is also a **cleansing day** only in **Week 1**.

In **Week 2** and **Week 3**, one **cleansing day** (Monday) is fine.

# Week 1 - Day 2

## *Fail-Safe Snacks*

These are your options:

- Spoonful of low fat yoghurt (I like French Vanilla the best)
- Sips of your simple smoothie
- Cup of vegetable or minestrone soup (always have a big bowl of vegetable soup in the fridge)
- A *few* sardines on a half slice of whole grain toast
- Half a banana squashed on a half slice of whole grain bread
- A few unsalted nuts (e.g. almonds, walnuts, soy nuts)
- A spoonful of hummus (chick peas) on a half slice of whole grain bread
- Half a small can of baked beans on a half slice of whole grain bread (pour off the sauce)

***Notes:***

If you just **have** to have some salt – buy some Potassium Salt called 'No Salt' and use just a little.

### Activity

| | |
|---|---|
| Walk - 25 min | ☐ |
| BAT exercises - Sets: 1 / Reps: 6 | ☐ |
| OUMs ... once | ☐ |

### Coping

| | | |
|---|---|---|
| Good sleep last night? | Yes | ☐ |
| Deep breathing? | Yes | ☐ |
| Laugh? | Yes | ☐ |
| Hug? | Yes | ☐ |
| Something good for someone else? | Yes | ☐ |
| Another 'thing' from the Relaxation List? | Yes | ☐ |

# Week 1 - Day 3

The Rule of 15 kicks in on Day 3 and each day thereafter.

Remember, 15 Plant Foods every day. Plant Foods are vegetables, fruits, nuts, seeds, grains. Little bits here and there – *small amounts*, not large amounts, e.g. three or four almonds, not three or four handfuls.

***Breakfast***

- Glass of water
- Fruit
- Grilled tomatoes on toast – whole grain bread e.g. soy & linseed bread
- Green tea/Jasmine tea

***Snack***

- Glass of water
- Equivalent of half a piece of fruit - half a banana or a few grapes
- Sip of soy milk or skim milk or smoothie
- Couple of rice crackers
- Coffee or tea OK

A snack is not necessarily **all** of these things.

***Lunch***

- Glass of water
- Bowl of vegetable soup or minestrone

***Alternative Lunch No. 1***

- Glass of water
- Sandwich – grain bread with one slice of cheese – three, four, five different salad ingredients

***Alternative Lunch No. 2***

- Glass of water
- Can of sardines or small can of salmon – pour off the oil
- Add some salad

***Alternative Lunch No. 3***

- Glass of water
- Salad bar

***Snack***

- Glass of water
- Same as morning snack

***Dinner***

- Grilled fish and lemon
- Three, four, five different vegetables
- Dessert – fruit sorbet
- A piece of chocolate if you wish (two squares)

The best fish are deep water and cold water fish. If you are eating lots of fish perhaps steer away from the large predators such as shark and swordfish, and go easy on the crustaceans and shell fish.
Remember the 2/3, 1/3 rule.
Remember The Rule of 15.
Remember that sardines also make a good snack (pour off the oil).

***Notes:***

You don't need butter or margarine – add just a teaspoon of olive oil.
Nuts should be unsalted. Buy some different seeds/pine nuts, macadamia nuts, olives etc. (keep them in little jars). These become alternative snacks.

# Week 1 - Day 3

***Tips***
These tips are attributed to Mr Rex Hunt, legendary fisherman and President of the highly successful **Fat Boys Club**.

1. Find some pieces of paper and write this on them ...
   **DON'T EAT CRAP**
   ... stick these notices around your house and in the office.
2. If you feel lousy in the first few days, then it's your bloody fault for eating all that muck before you started out on this Great Aussie journey.
3. If you're starting to think up excuses for giving this a miss, then you're as weak as the excuse.
4. My father dropped dead in his early 60s and you probably will too if you don't get your body in shape, inside and out.
5. I used to LIVE to EAT. Now I EAT to LIVE.
6. After two weeks of doing what Dr John told me to do, I felt fantastic. Are ***you*** fair dinkum, or not?

## Activity

| | |
|---|---|
| Take a nice walk if you wish | ☐ |

## Coping

| | | |
|---|---|---|
| Good sleep last night? | Yes | ☐ |
| Deep breathing? | Yes | ☐ |
| Laugh? | Yes | ☐ |
| Hug? | Yes | ☐ |
| Something good for someone else? | Yes | ☐ |
| Another 'thing' from the Relaxation List? | Yes | ☐ |

# Week 1 - Day 4

***Breakfast***
- Glass of water
- Fruit/ low fat yoghurt
- Grilled tomatoes on toast – whole grains e.g. soy and linseed bread
- Green tea or Jasmine Tea

***Snack***
- Glass of water
- Equivalent of half a piece of fruit half a banana or a few grapes
- Sip of soy milk or skim milk or smoothie or spoon of yoghurt
- Rice crackers or a few unsalted nuts
- Coffee or tea OK

***Lunch***
- Can of sardines or salmon – pour off the oil
- Salad

***Snack***
If you wish

***Dinner***
- Glass of water
- The best steak money can buy
- Three, four, five vegetables

***Notes:***
***Alternative Breakfast No. 2***
- Porridge – rolled oats (small bowl) – non-fat milk
- Fruit

Remember you don't need to eat all snacks at the same time – just enough to give your stomach something to do.

A piece of steak is 3 or 4 ozs (90 to 120 grams) – it doesn't cover the whole plate ... about the size of the palm of your hand.

## Activity

| | |
|---|---|
| Walk - 25 min | ☐ |
| BAT exercises - Sets: 1 / Reps: 6 | ☐ |
| OUMs ... once | ☐ |

## Coping

| | | |
|---|---|---|
| Good sleep last night? | Yes | ☐ |
| Deep breathing? | Yes | ☐ |
| Laugh? | Yes | ☐ |
| Hug? | Yes | ☐ |
| Something good for someone else? | Yes | ☐ |
| Another 'thing' from the Relaxation List? | Yes | ☐ |

# Week 1 - Day 5

***Breakfast***

- Glass of water
- Fruit
- Grilled tomatoes on toast – whole grains e.g. soy and linseed bread

***Snack***

You know the routine - same as Day 3

***Lunch***

- Glass of water
- Bowl of miso soup
- Salad Bar

***Snack***

- Glass of water etc. - same as Day 3

***Dinner***

- Glass of water
- Fish – vegetables as in Day 3

***Notes:***

In the three week **Switch On** periods, forget the pasta. Have some pasta in *your* two weeks for variety.

What is a salad bar? Well, find a place where you can self-serve or select what goes on your plate. Five, six, seven different things – not huge amounts (no dressings - except a touch of olive oil). You don't need huge amounts because you've had a bowl or cup of soup to start.

You should aim to eat four evening meals of fish each week. A canned sardine or salmon snack for lunch now and then is also good. If you absolutely, positively cannot eat fish, I feel sorry for you.

Maybe you weren't fed fish by your folks when you were a child. I don't know of any Italians, Greeks or Japanese who can't eat fish. If fish is definitely off your menu, replace it with skinless chicken breast, or very lean beef, lamb or pork.

## Activity

| Take a nice walk if you wish | ☐ ☐ ☐ |
| --- | --- |

## Coping

| | | |
| --- | --- | --- |
| Good sleep last night? | Yes | ☐ |
| Deep breathing? | Yes | ☐ |
| Laugh? | Yes | ☐ |
| Hug? | Yes | ☐ |
| Something good for someone else? | Yes | ☐ |
| Another 'thing' from the Relaxation List? | Yes | ☐ |

DID YOU GET YOUR 15 PLANT FOODS TODAY?

# Week 1 - Day 6

***Breakfast***

- Glass of water
- Fruit
- Two eggs – poached, boiled, fried (drain off the fat)
  Eat only 1/4 of the yolk and all the egg white (suggest you give the 3/4 of the yolk to your dog)

***Snack***

- Glass of water etc. – same as Day 3

***Lunch***

- Alternative No. 1, No. 2 or No. 3 – same as Day 3

***Snack***

- Glass of water etc. – same as Day 3

***Dinner***

- Glass of water
- Lamb chop or steak or how about some turkey?
- Three, four, five different vegetables
- Glass of wine or a piece of chocolate
- Dessert – fruit sorbet if you wish

***Notes:***

Why not go out to a restaurant tonight? Order steak or grilled fish and vegetables. If it doesn't come with vegetables because it doesn't say that on the menu – well then ask for vegetables ... please, thank you.

If you need an appetiser, order a salad (olive oil on the side) or a clear soup.

Please don't eat those luncheon meats or sliced chicken or turkey loaves (humans have interfered) – make sure it's the real thing.

If you eat chicken, do yourself a favour and throw away the skin. Chicken breast is best.

## Activity

| | |
|---|---|
| Walk - 25 min | ☐ |
| BAT exercises - Sets: 1 / Reps: 6 | ☐ |
| OUMs ... once | ☐ |

## Coping

| | | |
|---|---|---|
| Good sleep last night? | Yes | ☐ |
| Deep breathing? | Yes | ☐ |
| Laugh? | Yes | ☐ |
| Hug? | Yes | ☐ |
| Something good for someone else? | Yes | ☐ |
| Another 'thing' from the Relaxation List? | Yes | ☐ |

# Week 1 - Day 7

***Breakfast***
- Glass of water
- Fruit
- Two eggs – poached, boiled, fried (drain off the fat) – 1/4 of the yolk

***Snack***
- Glass of water etc. – same as Day 3

***Lunch***
- Glass of water
- Whatever you think is reasonable

***Snack***
- Glass of water etc. – same as Day 3

***Dinner***
- Glass of water
- Grilled fish and lemon
- Three, four, five different vegetables
- Glass of wine *or* a small piece of chocolate

***Notes:***

What did you say?

Wine **and** chocolate!

Give me a break – whose program is this?

I'm calling the shots in this three week period.

If you want wine **and** chocolate do that if you wish in your two weeks.

You can flip lunch and dinner any day you want to do this. That's what the mature Europeans do – a larger lunch, a siesta and then a small dinner.

## Activity

| | |
|---|---|
| Walk - 25 min | ☐ |
| BAT exercises - Sets: 1 / Reps: 6 | ☐ |
| OUMs ... once | ☐ |

## Coping

| | | |
|---|---|---|
| Good sleep last night? | Yes | ☐ |
| Deep breathing? | Yes | ☐ |
| Laugh? | Yes | ☐ |
| Hug? | Yes | ☐ |
| Something good for someone else? | Yes | ☐ |
| Another 'thing' from the Relaxation List? | Yes | ☐ |

# Dr John Tickell's 91 Day Success Chart

*At the completion of each week, transfer your weekly Livinglife points to the Scoreboard on the inside back cover*

## Week 2

| ACE | | M | T | W | T | F | S | S | My Total | Goal | Max |
|---|---|---|---|---|---|---|---|---|---|---|---|
| A1 | Did I do my walk today? | | | | | | | | | 14 | 14 |
| | 2 points per day – Goal: 14 points per week | | | | | | | | | | |
| | *If you walk minimum of 5 days per week – score 4 bonus points* | | | | | | | | | | |
| A2 | Did I do my strength work today? | | | | | | | | | 5 | 7 |
| | 1 point per day – Goal: 4 or 5 points per week | | | | | | | | | | |
| A3 | Did I do my OUMs today? | | | | | | | | | 5 | 7 |
| | 1 point per day – Goal: 4 or 5 points per week | | | | | | | | | | |
| | **ACTIVITY TOTALS** | | | | | | | | | **24** | **28** |
| | | M | T | W | T | F | S | S | | | |
| E1 | Did I eat/nibble my 15 Plant Foods today? | | | | | | | | | 12 | 14 |
| | 2 points per day – Goal: 12 points per week | | | | | | | | | | |
| E2 | Did I do the 2/3, 1/3 routine today? | | | | | | | | | 6 | 7 |
| | 1 point per day – Goal: 6 points per week | | | | | | | | | | |
| E3 | Did I eat breakfast today? | | | | | | | | | 6 | 7 |
| | 1 point per day – Goal: 6 points per week | | | | | | | | | | |
| | **EATING TOTALS** | | | | | | | | | **24** | **28** |
| | | M | T | W | T | F | S | S | | | |
| C1 | Did I have a laugh and give someone a hug today? | | | | | | | | | 6 | 7 |
| | 1 point per day – Goal: 6 points per week | | | | | | | | | | |
| C2 | Did I do some deep breathing and another relaxation thing today? | | | | | | | | | 6 | 7 |
| | 1 point per day – Goal: 6 points per week | | | | | | | | | | |
| C3 | Did I have a good sleep last night? | | | | | | | | | 6 | 7 |
| | 1 point per day – Goal: 6 points per week | | | | | | | | | | |
| C4 | Did I do something good for, or be nice to someone else today? | | | | | | | | | 6 | 7 |
| | 1 point per day – Goal: 6 points per week | | | | | | | | | | |
| | **COPING TOTALS** | | | | | | | | | **24** | **28** |
| | **WEEKLY GRAND TOTAL** | | | | | | | | | **72** | **84** |

*Switch-On weeks – aim at minimum of 60 LLPs per week*

*Switch-Off weeks – why not aim at the same number of LLPs?*

# Week 2 - Activity Schedule

Please mark these sessions in your diary - now - for this coming week.
Make the appointments with yourself.
The B.A.T and OUMs are laid out for you on Pages 143 and 150.

| | Monday Day 1 | Tuesday Day 2 | Wednesday Day 3 | Thursday Day 4 | Friday Day 5 | Saturday Day 6 | Sunday Day 7 |
|---|---|---|---|---|---|---|---|
| 1% | | Walk 25 min. | | Walk 25 min. | | Walk 25 min. | Walk 25 min. |
| SBW | | BAT Exercises Sets: 1 Reps: 8 | | BAT Exercises Sets: 1 Reps: 8 | | BAT Exercises Sets: 1 Reps: 8 | BAT Exercises Sets: 1 Reps: 8 |
| OUMs | | OUMs ...once | | OUMs ...once | | OUMs ...once | OUMs ...once |

# Week 2

***WEEK 2 is the same as WEEK 1***

Only DAY 1 is a day of **cleansing** (unless you wish to do two days of cleansing)

DAY 2 can be a repeat of DAY 3 or DAY 4 in WEEK 1.

Shoot for the Rule of 15 from DAY 2

***Notes:***

Have you been to the Asian market or supermarket? Have a browse. Did you know that you can buy real (frozen) soybeans? Try them as one of your vegetables this week and every week. They taste great.

## Activity

*Follow the Activity Schedule day by day*

| Activity | |
|---|---|
| Walk | ☐ |
| BAT | ☐ |
| OUMs | ☐ |

## Coping

*Each day fill out your weekly Success Chart*

| Coping | | |
|---|---|---|
| Good sleep last night? | Yes | ☐ |
| Deep breathing? | Yes | ☐ |
| Laugh? | Yes | ☐ |
| Hug? | Yes | ☐ |
| Something good for someone else? | Yes | ☐ |
| Another 'thing' from the Relaxation List? | Yes | ☐ |

# Dr John Tickell's 91 Day Success Chart

*At the completion of each week, transfer your weekly Livinglife points to the Scoreboard on the inside back cover*

| ACE | Week 3 | | Living*life* Points | | |
|---|---|---|---|---|---|
| | | M T W T F S S | My Total | Goal | Max |
| A1 | Did I do my walk today? | | | 14 | 14 |
| | 2 points per day – | Goal: 14 points per week | | | |
| | *If you walk minimum of 5 days per week – score 4 bonus points* | | | | |
| A2 | Did I do my strength work today? | | | 5 | 7 |
| | 1 point per day – | Goal: 4 or 5 points per week | | | |
| A3 | Did I do my OUMs today? | | | 5 | 7 |
| | 1 point per day – | Goal: 4 or 5 points per week | | | |
| | | **ACTIVITY TOTALS** | | **24** | **28** |
| | | M T W T F S S | | | |
| E1 | Did I eat/nibble my 15 Plant Foods today? | | | 12 | 14 |
| | 2 points per day – | Goal: 12 points per week | | | |
| E2 | Did I do the 2/3, 1/3 routine today? | | | 6 | 7 |
| | 1 point per day – | Goal: 6 points per week | | | |
| E3 | Did I eat breakfast today? | | | 6 | 7 |
| | 1 point per day – | Goal: 6 points per week | | | |
| | | **EATING TOTALS** | | **24** | **28** |
| | | M T W T F S S | | | |
| C1 | Did I have a laugh and give someone a hug today? | | | 6 | 7 |
| | 1 point per day – | Goal: 6 points per week | | | |
| C2 | Did I do some deep breathing and another relaxation thing today? | | | 6 | 7 |
| | 1 point per day – | Goal: 6 points per week | | | |
| C3 | Did I have a good sleep last night? | | | 6 | 7 |
| | 1 point per day – | Goal: 6 points per week | | | |
| C4 | Did I do something good for, or be nice to someone else today? | | | 6 | 7 |
| | 1 point per day – | Goal: 6 points per week | | | |
| | | **COPING TOTALS** | | **24** | **28** |
| | | **WEEKLY GRAND TOTAL** | | **72** | **84** |

*Switch-On weeks – aim at minimum of 60 LLPs per week*

*Switch-Off weeks – why not aim at the same number of LLPs?*

# Week 3 - Activity Schedule

Please mark these sessions in your diary - now - for this coming week.
Make the appointments with yourself.
The B.A.T and OUMs are laid out for you on Pages 143 and 150.

| | **Monday Day 1** | **Tuesday Day 2** | **Wednesday Day 3** | **Thursday Day4** | **Friday Day 5** | **Saturday Day 6** | **Sunday Day 7** |
|---|---|---|---|---|---|---|---|
| 1% | | Walk<br>25 mins. | | Walk<br>25 mins. | | Walk<br>25 mins. | Walk<br>25 mins. |
| SBW | | BAT<br>Exercises<br>Sets: 1<br>Reps: 10 | | BAT<br>Exercises<br>Sets: 1<br>Reps: 10 | | BAT<br>Exercises<br>Sets: 1<br>Reps: 10 | BAT<br>Exercises<br>Sets: 1<br>Reps: 10 |
| OUMs | | OUMs<br>… once | | OUMs<br>… once | | OUMs<br>… once | OUMs<br>… once |

# Week 3

***WEEK 3 is the same as WEEK 2***

You are settling into a routine of eating good whole foods now. Vary the fail-safe snacks – you don't need to do the same one every time.

Add some variety to your evening meal. Try an Asian stir-fry. Buy a wok, add a little high quality beef, lots of vegetables.

On DAY 3 add **one** egg for breakfast if you wish – ¼ of the yolk.

## Activity

*Follow the Activity Schedule day by day*

| Activity | ☐ |
|---|---|
| Walk | ☐ |
| BAT | ☐ |
| OUMs | ☐ |

## Coping

*Each day fill out your weekly Success Chart*

| Coping | | ☐ |
|---|---|---|
| Good sleep last night? | Yes | ☐ |
| Deep breathing? | Yes | ☐ |
| Laugh? | Yes | ☐ |
| Hug? | Yes | ☐ |
| Something good for someone else? | Yes | ☐ |
| Another 'thing' from the Relaxation List? | Yes | ☐ |

# Dr John Tickell's 91 Day Success Chart

*At the completion of each week, transfer your weekly Livinglife points to the Scoreboard on the inside back cover*

| ACE | Week 4 | M | T | W | T | F | S | S | My Total | Goal | Max |
|---|---|---|---|---|---|---|---|---|---|---|---|
| | | | | | | | | | | **Living*life* Points** | |
| A1 | Did I do my walk today? 2 points per day – Goal: 14 points per week. *If you walk minimum of 5 days per week – score 4 bonus points* | | | | | | | | | 14 | 14 |
| A2 | Did I do my strength work today? 1 point per day – Goal: 4 or 5 points per week | | | | | | | | | 5 | 7 |
| A3 | Did I do my OUMs today? 1 point per day – Goal: 4 or 5 points per week | | | | | | | | | 5 | 7 |
| | **ACTIVITY TOTALS** | | | | | | | | | 24 | 28 |
| E1 | Did I eat/nibble my 15 Plant Foods today? 2 points per day – Goal: 12 points per week | | | | | | | | | 12 | 14 |
| E2 | Did I do the 2/3, 1/3 routine today? 1 point per day – Goal: 6 points per week | | | | | | | | | 6 | 7 |
| E3 | Did I eat breakfast today? 1 point per day – Goal: 6 points per week | | | | | | | | | 6 | 7 |
| | **EATING TOTALS** | | | | | | | | | 24 | 28 |
| C1 | Did I have a laugh and give someone a hug today? 1 point per day – Goal: 6 points per week | | | | | | | | | 6 | 7 |
| C2 | Did I do some deep breathing and another relaxation thing today? 1 point per day – Goal: 6 points per week | | | | | | | | | 6 | 7 |
| C3 | Did I have a good sleep last night? 1 point per day – Goal: 6 points per week | | | | | | | | | 6 | 7 |
| C4 | Did I do something good for, or be nice to someone else today? 1 point per day – Goal: 6 points per week | | | | | | | | | 6 | 7 |
| | **COPING TOTALS** | | | | | | | | | 24 | 28 |
| | **WEEKLY GRAND TOTAL** | | | | | | | | | 72 | 84 |

*Switch-On weeks – aim at minimum of 60 LLPs per week*

*Switch-Off weeks – why not aim at the same number of LLPs?*

# Dr John Tickell's 91 Day Success Chart

*At the completion of each week, transfer your weekly Livinglife points to the Scoreboard on the inside back cover*

## Week 5

| ACE | | M | T | W | T | F | S | S | My Total | Goal | Max |
|---|---|---|---|---|---|---|---|---|---|---|---|
| A1 | Did I do my walk today? 2 points per day – Goal: 14 points per week. *If you walk minimum of 5 days per week – score 4 bonus points* | | | | | | | | | 14 | 14 |
| A2 | Did I do my strength work today? 1 point per day – Goal: 4 or 5 points per week | | | | | | | | | 5 | 7 |
| A3 | Did I do my OUMs today? 1 point per day – Goal: 4 or 5 points per week | | | | | | | | | 5 | 7 |
| | **ACTIVITY TOTALS** | | | | | | | | | **24** | **28** |
| | | M | T | W | T | F | S | S | | | |
| E1 | Did I eat/nibble my 15 Plant Foods today? 2 points per day – Goal: 12 points per week | | | | | | | | | 12 | 14 |
| E2 | Did I do the 2/3, 1/3 routine today? 1 point per day – Goal: 6 points per week | | | | | | | | | 6 | 7 |
| E3 | Did I eat breakfast today? 1 point per day – Goal: 6 points per week | | | | | | | | | 6 | 7 |
| | **EATING TOTALS** | | | | | | | | | **24** | **28** |
| | | M | T | W | T | F | S | S | | | |
| C1 | Did I have a laugh and give someone a hug today? 1 point per day – Goal: 6 points per week | | | | | | | | | 6 | 7 |
| C2 | Did I do some deep breathing and another relaxation thing today? 1 point per day – Goal: 6 points per week | | | | | | | | | 6 | 7 |
| C3 | Did I have a good sleep last night? 1 point per day – Goal: 6 points per week | | | | | | | | | 6 | 7 |
| C4 | Did I do something good for, or be nice to someone else today? 1 point per day – Goal: 6 points per week | | | | | | | | | 6 | 7 |
| | **COPING TOTALS** | | | | | | | | | **24** | **28** |
| | **WEEKLY GRAND TOTAL** | | | | | | | | | **72** | **84** |

*Switch-On weeks – aim at minimum of 60 LLPs per week*

*Switch-Off weeks – why not aim at the same number of LLPs?*

# Weeks 4 & 5 - Activity Schedule

Please mark these sessions in your diary - now - for this coming week.
Make the appointments with yourself.
The B.A.T and OUMs are laid out for you on Pages 143 and 150.

| | Monday Day 1 | Tuesday Day 2 | Wednesday Day 3 | Thursday Day4 | Friday Day 5 | Saturday Day 6 | Sunday Day 7 |
|---|---|---|---|---|---|---|---|
| 1% | | Walk | | Walk | | Walk | Walk |
| | | It's up to you... | | | | | |
| SBW | | BAT<br>Exercises<br>Sets:<br>Reps: | | BAT<br>Exercises<br>Sets:<br>Reps: | | BAT<br>Exercises<br>Sets:<br>Reps: | BAT<br>Exercises<br>Sets:<br>Reps: |
| | | It's up to you... | | | | | |
| OUMs | | OUMs<br>... once | | OUMs<br>... once | | OUMs<br>... once | OUMs<br>... once |
| | | It's up to you... | | | | | |

- In weeks 4 & 5, if you want to move it up a little, do so. It's your call.
- But you wouldn't do nothing and completely blow it, would you?

# Weeks 4 & 5

***Weeks 4 and 5 are the Hold weeks.***

I'm not going to advise you what to do day by day because you are basically on your own, but remember ...

- you would be crazy if you don't continue your exercise in these two weeks
- you would be crazy if you go stupid with your eating in these two weeks

Become a little innovative now. Go international.

From the Middle East – hummus, made with chickpeas. Buy it or do it yourself.

Asian – a stir fry once a week.

Italian – pasta, less refined is better, tomatoes, vegetables. And remember, non-fat Italians don't sit there eating huge bowls of pasta. If you eat lots of pasta, you get fat. It is **part** of an Italian meal, not just a giant Spaghetti Bolognese all by itself.

Rice – I forgot to mention that way over half the world's population eat rice **every** day, sometimes two and three times a day – and these guys aren't fat either. So if you want to introduce some whole grain rice, that's fine. It must be whole grain. Some people I know tell me you can't eat rice because it's carbohydrate, but around two and a half billion people seem to do fairly well with rice and vegetables and small amounts of protein.

If by some chance (in these two weeks) you put back half the weight you've lost, that's not good.

If you do, IMMEDIATELY begin WEEK 6.

## Activity

*Follow the Activity Schedule day by day*

| | |
|---|---|
| Walk | ☐ |
| BAT | ☐ |
| OUMs | ☐ |

## Coping

*Each day fill out your weekly Success Chart*

| | | |
|---|---|---|
| Good sleep last night? | Yes | ☐ |
| Deep breathing? | Yes | ☐ |
| Laugh? | Yes | ☐ |
| Hug? | Yes | ☐ |
| Something good for someone else? | Yes | ☐ |
| Another 'thing' from the Relaxation List? | Yes | ☐ |

# notes

## > Activity

At this stage of the game you are going to move for 1½% (one and a half percent) of your life. No big deal – you just do it! That's five half hours in a whole week.

The B.A.T. exercises and OUMs kick in for five little sessions each week.

## > Coping

A laugh, a hug, some deep breaths, another relaxation thing (have you 'done' some sunsets?) and be nice to someone else.

## > Eating

Let me ask you a question ...

*How fancy does your eating need to be?*

Are you a simple eater like me, or are you a real 'foodie' who needs to be reading about food, buying food and preparing food with lots of ideas and recipes to get your fix?

The challenge is this ...

Most people who love thinking about food and reading about food, eat too much of it.

Another question ...

*Do you like routine or do you become bored easily?*

In most aspects of my life, I need to be doing exciting things, discovering, planning and working out different ways to achieve.

However, when it comes to eating, if you announced to me that every day for the rest of my life I was going to have –

> The Same Breakfast

- Water
- Fruit and grains
- Grilled tomato and a couple of eggs now and then
- Green tea

> The Same Morning Break

- Café latté or low fat cappuccino
- A few nuts and seeds
- Sometimes a small piece of carrot cake

> The Same Lunch

- Bowl of minestrone and whole grain bread, or
- A great salad

> The Same Afternoon Snack

- Fruit, or
- Slice of whole grain bread with banana or asparagus or whatever, or
- Small can of sardines

> The Same Dinner

- Grilled fish and
- Lots of vegetables, and
- A glass or two of red wine

... would I be disappointed?

No way.

I'd love it.

So here we go with Week 6, Week 7 and Week 8 with a few 'recipes' to satisfy the foodies.

Remember this:

For overweight people, food is **THE** MAIN EVENT or at least **A** MAIN EVENT in their lives.

For normal weighted people, food is something you eat when you are **genuinely** hungry.

- You don't need huge servings, because you have fail-safe snacks to fall back on.
- You don't need second helpings, because the fail-safe snacks are always there.
- Drink a glass of water before each meal.

In the three week **Switch On** periods, you eat more carefully, similar to the way you thought about your meals in **Week 1, Week 2 and Week 3**.

Your snacks can include bits and pieces that help make up the 15 Plant Foods each day.

The learning process makes you become less dependent on being told **exactly** what to eat.

## Dr John Tickell's 91 Day Success Chart

*At the completion of each week, transfer your weekly Livinglife points to the Scoreboard on the inside back cover*

| ACE | Week 6 | M | T | W | T | F | S | S | My Total | Goal | Max |
|---|---|---|---|---|---|---|---|---|---|---|---|
| | | | | | | | | | **Livinglife Points** | | |
| A1 | Did I do my walk today? 2 points per day – Goal: 14 points per week. *If you walk minimum of 5 days per week – score 4 bonus points* | | | | | | | | | 14 | 14 |
| A2 | Did I do my strength work today? 1 point per day – Goal: 4 or 5 points per week | | | | | | | | | 5 | 7 |
| A3 | Did I do my OUMs today? 1 point per day – Goal: 4 or 5 points per week | | | | | | | | | 5 | 7 |
| | **ACTIVITY TOTALS** | | | | | | | | | **24** | **28** |
| E1 | Did I eat/nibble my 15 Plant Foods today? 2 points per day – Goal: 12 points per week | | | | | | | | | 12 | 14 |
| E2 | Did I do the 2/3, 1/3 routine today? 1 point per day – Goal: 6 points per week | | | | | | | | | 6 | 7 |
| E3 | Did I eat breakfast today? 1 point per day – Goal: 6 points per week | | | | | | | | | 6 | 7 |
| | **EATING TOTALS** | | | | | | | | | **24** | **28** |
| C1 | Did I have a laugh and give someone a hug today? 1 point per day – Goal: 6 points per week | | | | | | | | | 6 | 7 |
| C2 | Did I do some deep breathing and another relaxation thing today? 1 point per day – Goal: 6 points per week | | | | | | | | | 6 | 7 |
| C3 | Did I have a good sleep last night? 1 point per day – Goal: 6 points per week | | | | | | | | | 6 | 7 |
| C4 | Did I do something good for, or be nice to someone else today? 1 point per day – Goal: 6 points per week | | | | | | | | | 6 | 7 |
| | **COPING TOTALS** | | | | | | | | | **24** | **28** |
| | **WEEKLY GRAND TOTAL** | | | | | | | | | **72** | **84** |

*Switch-On weeks – aim at minimum of 60 LLPs per week*

*Switch-Off weeks – why not aim at the same number of LLPs?*

# Week 6 - Activity Schedule

Please mark these sessions in your diary - now - for this coming week.
Make the appointments with yourself.
The B.A.T and OUMs are laid out for you on Pages 143 and 150.

| | **Monday Day 1** | **Tuesday Day 2** | **Wednesday Day 3** | **Thursday Day 4** | **Friday Day 5** | **Saturday Day 6** | **Sunday Day 7** |
|---|---|---|---|---|---|---|---|
| 1.5% | | Walk 30 min. | Walk 30 min. | Walk 30 min. | | Walk 30 min. | Walk 30 min |
| SBW | | BAT Exercises Sets: 2 Reps: 6 | BAT Exercises Sets: 2 Reps: 6 | BAT Exercises Sets: 2 Reps: 6 | | BAT Exercises Sets: 2 Reps: 6 | BAT Excercises Sets: 2 Reps: 6 |
| OUMs | | OUMs … once | OUMs … once | OUMs … once | | OUMs … once | OUMs ... once |

- In week 6, move the walking periods up, so instead of one percent of your life, it's one and a half percent of your life. That's five days times 30 minutes = 150 minutes per week.
- If you are feeling good, do two sets of the BAT exercises some days or each exercise day. You go through the B exercises, then the A exercises, then the T exercises, then back to beginning and do them again.

# Week 6 - Day 1

***Breakfast***

- Glass of water
- Equivalent of one piece of fruit
- Grilled tomatoes
- Cup of green tea or Jasmine tea

***Snack***

- Glass of water
- Equivalent of half a piece of fruit - half a banana or a few grapes
- Sip of soy milk or skim milk smoothie
- Coffee or tea OK
- Check out the Fail-Safe Snack list again

***Lunch***

- Glass of water
- Bowl of vegetable soup or minestrone with a little low fat grated cheese

***Snack***

- Glass of water etc.

***Dinner***

- Glass of water
- Bowl of vegetable soup or minestrone (grated cheese is optional)

***Evening Snack or Get Up During the Night Snack***

- Two spoons of low fat yoghurt
- Sip of smoothie, soy milk/skim milk, or
- Cup of minestrone

***Notes:***

Day 1 is a **Cleansing Day.**

Go back to Week 1 Day 1 and re-read the notes.

The use of pepper on your grilled tomatoes and minestrone is fine.

## Activity

| Gentle or brisk walk if you wish | ☐ |
|---|---|

## Coping

| | | |
|---|---|---|
| Good sleep last night? | Yes | ☐ |
| Deep breathing? | Yes | ☐ |
| Laugh? | Yes | ☐ |
| Hug? | Yes | ☐ |
| Something good for someone else? | Yes | ☐ |
| Another 'thing' from the Relaxation List? | Yes | ☐ |

# Week 6 - Day 2

***Day 2 is the same as Day 1***

Day 2 is also a **Cleansing Day** only in Week 6.

In Week 7 and Week 8, one **Cleansing Day** (Monday) is fine.

## *Fail-safe snacks*

These are your options:

- Spoonful of low fat yoghurt (I like French Vanilla the best)
- Sips of your simple smoothie
- Cup of vegetable or minestrone soup (always have a big bowl of vegetable. soup in the fridge)
- A *few* sardines on half slice of whole grain toast
- Half a banana squashed on a half slice of whole grain bread
- A few unsalted nuts (e.g. almonds, walnuts, soy nuts)
- A spoonful of hummus (chick peas) on a half slice of whole grain bread
- Half a small can of baked beans on a half slice of whole grain bread (pour off the sauce)

### Activity

| | |
|---|---|
| Walk - 30 min | ☐ |
| BAT exercises - Sets: 2 / Reps: 6 | ☐ |
| OUMs ... once | ☐ |

### Coping

| | | |
|---|---|---|
| Good sleep last night? | Yes | ☐ |
| Deep breathing? | Yes | ☐ |
| Laugh? | Yes | ☐ |
| Hug? | Yes | ☐ |
| Something good for someone else? | Yes | ☐ |
| Another 'thing' from the Relaxation List? | Yes | ☐ |

# Week 6 - Day 3

The Rule of 15 is back in town.

Remember, 15 Plant Foods every day.

Plant Foods are vegetables, fruits, nuts, seeds, grains.

Little bits here and there - small amounts, not large amounts. e.g. three or four almonds, walnuts etc., not three or four handfuls.

***Breakfast***

- Glass of water
- Fruit
- Muesli Mix* or a Weetbix/ Vitabrits
- Eggs twice a week – you can have your Saturday eggs today if you wish (1/4 of the yolk)
- Green Tea or Jasmine Tea

***Snack***

- Fruit, smoothie, rice crackers
- Take it easy

***Lunch***

- The 'S' Routine - i.e ... Soup or Sandwich or Salad or Sardines or Salmon, or see Alternative Lunches Week 1 Day 3

***Dinner***

- Fish and vegetables*

***Dessert***

- Fruit sorbet

***Notes:***

On Days 3, 5 and 7, forget the tomatoes on toast and have a little muesli mix with your fruit.

* See Recipe Section - Page 239

## Activity

| | |
|---|---|
| Walk - 30 min | ☐ |
| BAT exercises - Sets: 2 / Reps: 6 | ☐ |
| OUMs ... once | ☐ |

## Coping

| | | |
|---|---|---|
| Good sleep last night? | Yes | ☐ |
| Deep breathing? | Yes | ☐ |
| Laugh? | Yes | ☐ |
| Hug? | Yes | ☐ |
| Something good for someone else? | Yes | ☐ |
| Another 'thing' from the Relaxation List? | Yes | ☐ |

# Week 6 - Day 4

***Breakfast***
- Fruit
- Grilled tomatoes on toast

***Snacks***
- As per usual

***Lunch***
- The 'S' routine ...

***Dinner***
- Steak and vegetables
  (Kangaroo if you're fair dinkum)

***Notes:***
A piece of steak for human consumption is 3 to 4 ounces (90 to 120 grams) - it doesn't cover the whole plate.

## Activity

| | |
|---|---|
| Walk - 30 min | ☐ |
| BAT exercises - Sets: 2 / Reps: 6 | ☐ |
| OUMs ... once | ☐ |

## Coping

| | | |
|---|---|---|
| Good sleep last night? | Yes | ☐ |
| Deep breathing? | Yes | ☐ |
| Laugh? | Yes | ☐ |
| Hug? | Yes | ☐ |
| Something good for someone else? | Yes | ☐ |
| Another 'thing' from the Relaxation List? | Yes | ☐ |

# Week 6 - Day 5

***Breakfast***

- Fruit and muesli

***Lunch***

- The 'S' routine ...

***Dinner***

- Fish and vegetables

***Notes:***

Keep your little snack jars topped up with seeds, nuts, olives etc.

***Remember the Rule of 15***

## Activity

| It's up to you | ☐ |
|---|---|

## Coping

| | | |
|---|---|---|
| Good sleep last night? | Yes | ☐ |
| Deep breathing? | Yes | ☐ |
| Laugh? | Yes | ☐ |
| Hug? | Yes | ☐ |
| Something good for someone else? | Yes | ☐ |
| Another 'thing' from the Relaxation List? | Yes | ☐ |

# Week 6 - Day 6

Suggestion – prepare a vegetable casserole* for the weekend

***Breakfast***

- Fruit
- Two eggs, mushrooms, tomato

***Lunch***

- The 'S' routine or vegetable casserole

***Dinner***

- Lamb chops, or chicken* or turkey or kangaroo
- Vegetables
- Glass of wine
- Dessert - fruit sorbet or fruit and some low fat yoghurt

***Notes:***

Try the egg white omelette* for a change - add a ¼ of the yolk if you wish

Day 6 is a Restaurant Night (or Day 5 or Day 7).

* See Recipe section - page 239

## Activity

| | |
|---|---|
| Walk - 30 min | ☐ |
| BAT exercises - Sets: 2 / Reps: 6 | ☐ |
| OUMs ... once | ☐ |

## Coping

| | | |
|---|---|---|
| Good sleep last night? | Yes | ☐ |
| Deep breathing? | Yes | ☐ |
| Laugh? | Yes | ☐ |
| Hug? | Yes | ☐ |
| Something good for someone else? | Yes | ☐ |
| Another 'thing' from the Relaxation List? | Yes | ☐ |

# Week 6 - Day 7

***Breakfast***
- Fruit and muesli
- Two eggs on grain toast (all the egg whites and ¼ of the yolks)

***Lunch***
- The 'S' Routine - or another 'S' - Spaghetti (small serve) with tomato, mushrooms and basil

***Dinner***
- Fish and vegetables
- Glass of wine
- Fruit dessert and a chocolate

***Notes:***

Remember: The Rule of 15
2/3 - 1/3

You can flip lunch and dinner any day you want to do this. That's what the mature Europeans do – a larger lunch, a siesta and then a small dinner.

## Activity

| | |
|---|---|
| Walk - 30 min | ☐ |
| BAT exercises - Sets: 2 / Reps: 6 | ☐ |
| OUMs ... once | ☐ |

## Coping

| | | |
|---|---|---|
| Good sleep last night? | Yes | ☐ |
| Deep breathing? | Yes | ☐ |
| Laugh? | Yes | ☐ |
| Hug? | Yes | ☐ |
| Something good for someone else? | Yes | ☐ |
| Another 'thing' from the Relaxation List? | Yes | ☐ |

# Dr John Tickell's 91 Day Success Chart

*At the completion of each week, transfer your weekly Livinglife points to the Scoreboard on the inside back cover*

| ACE | Week 7 | M | T | W | T | F | S | S | My Total | Goal | Max |
|---|---|---|---|---|---|---|---|---|---|---|---|
| | | | | | | | | | | **Living*life* Points** | |
| A1 | Did I do my walk today? 2 points per day – Goal: 14 points per week. *If you walk minimum of 5 days per week – score 4 bonus points* | | | | | | | | | 14 | 14 |
| A2 | Did I do my strength work today? 1 point per day – Goal: 4 or 5 points per week | | | | | | | | | 5 | 7 |
| A3 | Did I do my OUMs today? 1 point per day – Goal: 4 or 5 points per week | | | | | | | | | 5 | 7 |
| | **ACTIVITY TOTALS** | | | | | | | | | **24** | **28** |
| E1 | Did I eat/nibble my 15 Plant Foods today? 2 points per day – Goal: 12 points per week | | | | | | | | | 12 | 14 |
| E2 | Did I do the 2/3, 1/3 routine today? 1 point per day – Goal: 6 points per week | | | | | | | | | 6 | 7 |
| E3 | Did I eat breakfast today? 1 point per day – Goal: 6 points per week | | | | | | | | | 6 | 7 |
| | **EATING TOTALS** | | | | | | | | | **24** | **28** |
| C1 | Did I have a laugh and give someone a hug today? 1 point per day – Goal: 6 points per week | | | | | | | | | 6 | 7 |
| C2 | Did I do some deep breathing and another relaxation thing today? 1 point per day – Goal: 6 points per week | | | | | | | | | 6 | 7 |
| C3 | Did I have a good sleep last night? 1 point per day – Goal: 6 points per week | | | | | | | | | 6 | 7 |
| C4 | Did I do something good for, or be nice to someone else today? 1 point per day – Goal: 6 points per week | | | | | | | | | 6 | 7 |
| | **COPING TOTALS** | | | | | | | | | **24** | **28** |
| | **WEEKLY GRAND TOTAL** | | | | | | | | | **72** | **84** |

*Switch-On weeks – aim at minimum of 60 LLPs per week*

*Switch-Off weeks – why not aim at the same number of LLPs?*

# Week 7 - Activity Schedule

Please mark these sessions in your diary - now - for this coming week.
Make the appointments with yourself.
The B.A.T and OUMs are laid out for you on Pages 143 and 150.

| | Monday Day 1 | Tuesday Day 2 | Wednesday Day 3 | Thursday Day 4 | Friday Day 5 | Saturday Day 6 | Sunday Day 7 |
|---|---|---|---|---|---|---|---|
| 1.5% | | Walk 30 min. | Walk 30 min. | Walk 30 min. | | Walk 30 min. | Walk 30 min |
| SBW | | BAT Exercises Sets: 2 Reps: 8 | BAT Exercises Sets: 2 Reps: 8 | BAT Exercises Sets: 2 Reps: 8 | | BAT Exercises Sets: 2 Reps: 8 | BAT Excercises Sets: 2 Reps: 8 |
| OUMs | | OUMs ... once | OUMs ... once | OUMs ... once | | OUMs ... once | OUMs ... once |

# Week 7

***WEEK 7 is the same as WEEK 6***

Only one day of **cleansing** and you are shooting for The Rule of 15 each day.

***Something to think about ...***

That junk you used to eat ... you will get to a stage (and maybe you're there already) where if you absolutely must have a chocolate bar or hamburger or fries or a bag of chips or fried chicken or some salami, then have a crack at it but don't eat the whole thing!

If I am served 300 fries on a plate in a restaurant, I can eat three and walk away from the other 297.

What is the point in eating them all? A billion calories and lots of fat - that's the point! You're only feeding your tongue - the rest of your body doesn't want them.

I visualise all that fat sludging up the tiny coronary arteries (the ones that keep your heart alive) that are the width of **one-fifth** of your little finger.

If I'm starving to death in an American Airport, I've been known to grab a burger, take two bites, then throw the rest in the trash.

It's a game - the game of life!

## Activity

*Follow the Activity Schedule day by day*

| | |
|---|---|
| Walk | ☐ |
| BAT | ☐ |
| OUMs | ☐ |

## Coping

*Each day fill out your weekly Success Chart*

| | | |
|---|---|---|
| Good sleep last night? | Yes | ☐ |
| Deep breathing? | Yes | ☐ |
| Laugh? | Yes | ☐ |
| Hug? | Yes | ☐ |
| Something good for someone else? | Yes | ☐ |
| Another 'thing' from the Relaxation List? | Yes | ☐ |

# Dr John Tickell's 91 Day Success Chart

*At the completion of each week, transfer your weekly Livinglife points to the Scoreboard on the inside back cover*

| ACE | Week 8 | M | T | W | T | F | S | S | My Total | Goal | Max |
|---|---|---|---|---|---|---|---|---|---|---|---|
| | | | | | | | | | **Living*life* Points** | | |
| A1 | Did I do my walk today? 2 points per day – Goal: 14 points per week. *If you walk minimum of 5 days per week – score 4 bonus points* | | | | | | | | | 14 | 14 |
| A2 | Did I do my strength work today? 1 point per day – Goal: 4 or 5 points per week | | | | | | | | | 5 | 7 |
| A3 | Did I do my OUMs today? 1 point per day – Goal: 4 or 5 points per week | | | | | | | | | 5 | 7 |
| | **ACTIVITY TOTALS** | | | | | | | | | **24** | **28** |
| E1 | Did I eat/nibble my 15 Plant Foods today? 2 points per day – Goal: 12 points per week | | | | | | | | | 12 | 14 |
| E2 | Did I do the 2/3, 1/3 routine today? 1 point per day – Goal: 6 points per week | | | | | | | | | 6 | 7 |
| E3 | Did I eat breakfast today? 1 point per day – Goal: 6 points per week | | | | | | | | | 6 | 7 |
| | **EATING TOTALS** | | | | | | | | | **24** | **28** |
| C1 | Did I have a laugh and give someone a hug today? 1 point per day – Goal: 6 points per week | | | | | | | | | 6 | 7 |
| C2 | Did I do some deep breathing and another relaxation thing today? 1 point per day – Goal: 6 points per week | | | | | | | | | 6 | 7 |
| C3 | Did I have a good sleep last night? 1 point per day – Goal: 6 points per week | | | | | | | | | 6 | 7 |
| C4 | Did I do something good for, or be nice to someone else today? 1 point per day – Goal: 6 points per week | | | | | | | | | 6 | 7 |
| | **COPING TOTALS** | | | | | | | | | **24** | **28** |
| | **WEEKLY GRAND TOTAL** | | | | | | | | | **72** | **84** |

*Switch-On weeks – aim at minimum of 60 LLPs per week*

*Switch-Off weeks – why not aim at the same number of LLPs?*

# Week 8 - Activity Schedule

Please mark these sessions in your diary - now - for this coming week.
Make the appointments with yourself.
The B.A.T and OUMs are laid out for you on Pages 143 and 150.

| | Monday Day 1 | Tuesday Day 2 | Wednesday Day 3 | Thursday Day 4 | Friday Day 5 | Saturday Day 6 | Sunday Day 7 |
|---|---|---|---|---|---|---|---|
| 1.5% | | Walk 30 min. | Walk 30 min. | Walk 30 min. | | Walk 30 min. | Walk 30 min |
| SBW | | BAT Exercises Sets: 2 Reps: 10 | BAT Exercises Sets: 2 Reps: 10 | BAT Exercises Sets: 2 Reps: 10 | | BAT Exercises Sets: 2 Reps: 10 | BAT Excercises Sets: 2 Reps: 10 |
| OUMs | | OUMs ... once | OUMs ... once | OUMs ... once | | OUMs ... once | OUMs ... once |

# Week 8

***WEEK 8 is the same as WEEK 7***

Continue The Rule of 15 each day

## *'Going Well'*

*Follow the Activity Schedule day by day*

### Activity

| Activity | |
|---|---|
| Walk | ☐ |
| BAT | ☐ |
| OUMs | ☐ |

*Each day fill out your weekly Success Chart*

### Coping

| Coping | | |
|---|---|---|
| Good sleep last night? | Yes | ☐ |
| Deep breathing? | Yes | ☐ |
| Laugh? | Yes | ☐ |
| Hug? | Yes | ☐ |
| Something good for someone else? | Yes | ☐ |
| Another 'thing' from the Relaxation List? | Yes | ☐ |

# Dr John Tickell's 91 Day Success Chart

*At the completion of each week, transfer your weekly Livinglife points to the Scoreboard on the inside back cover*

| ACE | Week 9 | M | T | W | T | F | S | S | My Total | Goal | Max |
|---|---|---|---|---|---|---|---|---|---|---|---|
| | | | | | | | | | **Living*life* Points** | | |
| A1 | Did I do my walk today?<br>2 points per day – Goal: 14 points per week<br>*If you walk minimum of 5 days per week – score 4 bonus points* | | | | | | | | | 14 | 14 |
| A2 | Did I do my strength work today?<br>1 point per day – Goal: 4 or 5 points per week | | | | | | | | | 5 | 7 |
| A3 | Did I do my OUMs today?<br>1 point per day – Goal: 4 or 5 points per week | | | | | | | | | 5 | 7 |
| | **ACTIVITY TOTALS** | | | | | | | | | **24** | **28** |
| | | M | T | W | T | F | S | S | | | |
| E1 | Did I eat/nibble my 15 Plant Foods today?<br>2 points per day – Goal: 12 points per week | | | | | | | | | 12 | 14 |
| E2 | Did I do the 2/3, 1/3 routine today?<br>1 point per day – Goal: 6 points per week | | | | | | | | | 6 | 7 |
| E3 | Did I eat breakfast today?<br>1 point per day – Goal: 6 points per week | | | | | | | | | 6 | 7 |
| | **EATING TOTALS** | | | | | | | | | **24** | **28** |
| | | M | T | W | T | F | S | S | | | |
| C1 | Did I have a laugh and give someone a hug today?<br>1 point per day – Goal: 6 points per week | | | | | | | | | 6 | 7 |
| C2 | Did I do some deep breathing and another relaxation thing today?<br>1 point per day – Goal: 6 points per week | | | | | | | | | 6 | 7 |
| C3 | Did I have a good sleep last night?<br>1 point per day – Goal: 6 points per week | | | | | | | | | 6 | 7 |
| C4 | Did I do something good for, or be nice to someone else today?<br>1 point per day – Goal: 6 points per week | | | | | | | | | 6 | 7 |
| | **COPING TOTALS** | | | | | | | | | **24** | **28** |
| | **WEEKLY GRAND TOTAL** | | | | | | | | | **72** | **84** |

*Switch-On weeks – aim at minimum of 60 LLPs per week*

*Switch-Off weeks – why not aim at the same number of LLPs?*

# Dr John Tickell's 91 Day Success Chart

*At the completion of each week, transfer your weekly Livinglife points to the Scoreboard on the inside back cover*

| ACE | Week 10 | M | T | W | T | F | S | S | My Total | Goal | Max |
|---|---|---|---|---|---|---|---|---|---|---|---|
| | | | | | | | | | Living*life* Points | | |
| A1 | Did I do my walk today? 2 points per day – Goal: 14 points per week | | | | | | | | | 14 | 14 |
| | *If you walk minimum of 5 days per week – score 4 bonus points* | | | | | | | | | | |
| A2 | Did I do my strength work today? 1 point per day – Goal: 4 or 5 points per week | | | | | | | | | 5 | 7 |
| A3 | Did I do my OUMs today? 1 point per day – Goal: 4 or 5 points per week | | | | | | | | | 5 | 7 |
| | **ACTIVITY TOTALS** | | | | | | | | | **24** | **28** |
| E1 | Did I eat/nibble my 15 Plant Foods today? 2 points per day – Goal: 12 points per week | | | | | | | | | 12 | 14 |
| E2 | Did I do the 2/3, 1/3 routine today? 1 point per day – Goal: 6 points per week | | | | | | | | | 6 | 7 |
| E3 | Did I eat breakfast today? 1 point per day – Goal: 6 points per week | | | | | | | | | 6 | 7 |
| | **EATING TOTALS** | | | | | | | | | **24** | **28** |
| C1 | Did I have a laugh and give someone a hug today? 1 point per day – Goal: 6 points per week | | | | | | | | | 6 | 7 |
| C2 | Did I do some deep breathing and another relaxation thing today? 1 point per day – Goal: 6 points per week | | | | | | | | | 6 | 7 |
| C3 | Did I have a good sleep last night? 1 point per day – Goal: 6 points per week | | | | | | | | | 6 | 7 |
| C4 | Did I do something good for, or be nice to someone else today? 1 point per day – Goal: 6 points per week | | | | | | | | | 6 | 7 |
| | **COPING TOTALS** | | | | | | | | | **24** | **28** |
| | **WEEKLY GRAND TOTAL** | | | | | | | | | **72** | **84** |

*Switch-On weeks – aim at minimum of 60 LLPs per week*

*Switch-Off weeks – why not aim at the same number of LLPs?*

# Weeks 9 & 10 - Activity Schedule

Please mark these sessions in your diary - now - for this coming week.
Make the appointments with yourself.
The B.A.T and OUMs are laid out for you on Pages 143 and 150.

| | Monday Day 1 | Tuesday Day 2 | Wednesday Day 3 | Thursday Day 4 | Friday Day 5 | Saturday Day 6 | Sunday Day 7 |
|---|---|---|---|---|---|---|---|
| | | Walk | Walk | Walk | | Walk | Walk |
| It's up to you ... | | | | | | | |
| SBW | | BAT Exercises Sets: Reps: | BAT Exercises Sets: Reps: | BAT Exercises Sets: Reps: | | BAT Exercises Sets: Reps: | BAT Exercises Sets: Reps: |
| It's up to you... | | | | | | | |
| OUMs | | OUMs ... once | OUMs ... once | OUMs ... once | | OUMs ... once | OUMs ... once |
| It's up to you ... | | | | | | | |

# Weeks 9 & 10

***These are Hold weeks***

Don't let yourself down – 'steady as she goes'.

Remember that list of foods called WHY WOULD YOU EAT THEM?

Check them out and see if there is something there that gets you really excited.

By now, you probably won't be all that turned on by them, but if you want to have a go, you only need a little. Otherwise you are just feeding your tongue and what's the point in doing that?

A small scoop of low fat ice cream instead of two or three chunks. That's OK.

# Dr John Tickell's 91 Day Success Chart

*At the completion of each week, transfer your weekly Livinglife points to the Scoreboard on the inside back cover*

## ACE — Week 11

| | | M | T | W | T | F | S | S | My Total | Goal | Max |
|---|---|---|---|---|---|---|---|---|---|---|---|
| | | | | | | | | | | *Livinglife Points* | |
| A1 | Did I do my walk today? 2 points per day – Goal: 14 points per week. *If you walk minimum of 5 days per week – score 4 bonus points* | | | | | | | | | 14 | 14 |
| A2 | Did I do my strength work today? 1 point per day – Goal: 4 or 5 points per week | | | | | | | | | 5 | 7 |
| A3 | Did I do my OUMs today? 1 point per day – Goal: 4 or 5 points per week | | | | | | | | | 5 | 7 |
| | **ACTIVITY TOTALS** | | | | | | | | | **24** | **28** |
| E1 | Did I eat/nibble my 15 Plant Foods today? 2 points per day – Goal: 12 points per week | | | | | | | | | 12 | 14 |
| E2 | Did I do the 2/3, 1/3 routine today? 1 point per day – Goal: 6 points per week | | | | | | | | | 6 | 7 |
| E3 | Did I eat breakfast today? 1 point per day – Goal: 6 points per week | | | | | | | | | 6 | 7 |
| | **EATING TOTALS** | | | | | | | | | **24** | **28** |
| C1 | Did I have a laugh and give someone a hug today? 1 point per day – Goal: 6 points per week | | | | | | | | | 6 | 7 |
| C2 | Did I do some deep breathing and another relaxation thing today? 1 point per day – Goal: 6 points per week | | | | | | | | | 6 | 7 |
| C3 | Did I have a good sleep last night? 1 point per day – Goal: 6 points per week | | | | | | | | | 6 | 7 |
| C4 | Did I do something good for, or be nice to someone else today? 1 point per day – Goal: 6 points per week | | | | | | | | | 6 | 7 |
| | **COPING TOTALS** | | | | | | | | | **24** | **28** |
| | **WEEKLY GRAND TOTAL** | | | | | | | | | **72** | **84** |

*Switch-On weeks – aim at minimum of 60 LLPs per week*

*Switch-Off weeks – why not aim at the same number of LLPs?*

# Week 11 - Activity Schedule

Please mark these sessions in your diary - now - for this coming week.
Make the appointments with yourself.
The B.A.T and OUMs are laid out for you on Pages 143 and 150.

| | Monday Day 1 | Tuesday Day 2 | Wednesday Day 3 | Thursday Day 4 | Friday Day 5 | Saturday Day 6 | Sunday Day 7 |
|---|---|---|---|---|---|---|---|
| 1.5% | | Walk<br>30 min. | Walk<br>30 min. | Walk<br>30 min. | | Walk<br>30 min. | Walk<br>30 min |
| SBW | | BAT<br>Exercises<br>Sets: 2<br>Reps: 6 | BAT<br>Exercises<br>Sets: 2<br>Reps: 6 | BAT<br>Exercises<br>Sets: 2<br>Reps: 6 | | BAT<br>Exercises<br>Sets: 2<br>Reps: 6 | BAT<br>Excercises<br>Sets: 2<br>Reps: 6 |
| OUMs | | OUMs<br>... once | OUMs<br>... once | OUMs<br>... once | | OUMs<br>... once | OUMs<br>... once |

- In week 11, if you are feeling good, you can use weights that are a touch heavier.

# Week 11 - Day 1

***Breakfast***

- Glass of water
- Equivalent of one piece of fruit only e.g. half a banana, half an apple, or a few grapes, three or four prunes, etc.
- Grilled tomatoes - no salt - no bread - no toast
- Cup of green tea or Jasmine tea

***Snack***

- Glass of water
- Equivalent of half a piece of fruit - half a banana or a few grapes
- Sip of soy milk or skim milk smoothie
- Coffee or tea OK
- Check out the Fail-Safe Snack list again.

***Lunch***

- Glass of water
- Bowl of vegetable soup or minestrone with a little low fat grated cheese

***Snack***

- Glass of water etc.

***Dinner***

- Glass of water
- Bowl of vegetable soup or minestrone (grated cheese is optional)

***Evening Snack or Get Up During the Night Snack***

- Two spoons of low fat yoghurt
- Sip of smoothie, soy milk/skim milk or
- Cup of minestrone

***Notes:***

Day 1 is a **cleansing day**

Please read the Week 1 - Day 1 notes again.

The use of pepper on your grilled tomatoes and minestrone is fine.

# Week 11 - Days 2-7

***Breakfast***

Today and **EVERY DAY**

Are you OK with fruit, tomatoes, an egg or eggs now and then, muesli or a weetbix here and there?

Or maybe some rolled oats porridge with low fat milk and maybe some fruit?

I've been doing that for 50 years, and I'm not bored, but if you're desperate to light up your life, you may try (as an alternative) –

- Avocado and tomato on whole grain toast
- Smoked salmon, or
- Book into an Asian Hotel for breakfast and give it a go (you won't need lunch)

***Lunch***

Today and **EVERY DAY**

- A glass of water before every meal
- The 'S' Routine sounds good to me

  Soup or Sandwich (wholegrain – try soy and linseed bread) or Salad or Sardines or Salmon (Tuna is fine).

***Dinner***

Today and **EVERY DAY**

- A glass of water before the evening meal
- The Two-Thirds, One-Third Rule is uppermost in our minds
- Dinner is 2/3 BASIC – plant – vegetables – and the rest of your plate can be fish, high quality beef, veal, lamb, kangaroo or chicken breast

  At home, Sue would prepare between six and ten different vegetables each evening. When people come to dinner at our home, they can't believe all the trouble she has gone to.

  But Sue says – *'It's no trouble, in fact, way less work than preparing some fancy recipe for the meal'.*

  Good point.

  And, we are not talking about a huge amount of food here – small portions, larger variety. That's the name of the game.

  In a Western restaurant, because they have absolutely no idea of the 2/3, l/3 concept, I generally request mixed steamed vegetables as a side order to the main meal. That's if I haven't ordered roasted vegetables as an appetiser.

- Another trick. If you are worried you may overeat at a restaurant, then have a bowl of minestrone **before** you leave home!

***Dessert***

In a restaurant, there are no *Great Australian Diet* desserts (except fruit), so you may wish to have a fling. If you do, order one dessert and four spoons and split the 'thing' four ways. That's all you need.

# Week 11 - Days 2-7

***Notes:***

- You don't need large portions or servings because you think you might get hungry 'later on'. The Fail-Safe Snacks will take care of later on.
- Switch dinner and lunch if you wish, but there is absolutely no point in having **two** large cooked meals in the one day.
- You can flip lunch and dinner any day you want to do this. That's what the mature Europeans do – a larger lunch, a siesta and then a small dinner.

# Dr John Tickell's 91 Day Success Chart

*At the completion of each week, transfer your weekly Livinglife points to the Scoreboard on the inside back cover*

## Week 12

| ACE | | M T W T F S S | My Total | Goal | Max |
|---|---|---|---|---|---|
| A1 | Did I do my walk today? 2 points per day – | Goal: 14 points per week | | 14 | 14 |
| | *If you walk minimum of 5 days per week – score 4 bonus points* | | | | |
| A2 | Did I do my strength work today? 1 point per day – | Goal: 4 or 5 points per week | | 5 | 7 |
| A3 | Did I do my OUMs today? 1 point per day – | Goal: 4 or 5 points per week | | 5 | 7 |
| | | **ACTIVITY TOTALS** | | **24** | **28** |
| E1 | Did I eat/nibble my 15 Plant Foods today? 2 points per day – | Goal: 12 points per week | | 12 | 14 |
| E2 | Did I do the 2/3, 1/3 routine today? 1 point per day – | Goal: 6 points per week | | 6 | 7 |
| E3 | Did I eat breakfast today? 1 point per day – | Goal: 6 points per week | | 6 | 7 |
| | | **EATING TOTALS** | | **24** | **28** |
| C1 | Did I have a laugh and give someone a hug today? 1 point per day – | Goal: 6 points per week | | 6 | 7 |
| C2 | Did I do some deep breathing and another relaxation thing today? 1 point per day – | Goal: 6 points per week | | 6 | 7 |
| C3 | Did I have a good sleep last night? 1 point per day – | Goal: 6 points per week | | 6 | 7 |
| C4 | Did I do something good for, or be nice to someone else today? 1 point per day – | Goal: 6 points per week | | 6 | 7 |
| | | **COPING TOTALS** | | **24** | **28** |
| | | **WEEKLY GRAND TOTAL** | | **72** | **84** |

*Switch-On weeks – aim at minimum of 60 LLPs per week*

*Switch-Off weeks – why not aim at the same number of LLPs?*

# Week 12 - Activity Schedule

Please mark these sessions in your diary - now - for this coming week.
Make the appointments with yourself.
The B.A.T and OUMs are laid out for you on Pages 143 and 150.

| | Monday Day 1 | Tuesday Day 2 | Wednesday Day 3 | Thursday Day 4 | Friday Day 5 | Saturday Day 6 | Sunday Day 7 |
|---|---|---|---|---|---|---|---|
| 1.5% | | Walk 30 min. | Walk 30 min. | Walk 30 mins. | | Walk 30 min. | Walk 30 min |
| SBW | | BAT Exercises Sets: 2 Reps: 8 | BAT Exercises Sets: 2 Reps: 8 | BAT Exercises Sets: 2 Reps: 8 | | BAT Exercises Sets: 2 Reps: 8 | BAT Excercises Sets: 2 Reps: 8 |
| OUMs | | OUMs ... once | OUMs ... once | OUMs ... once | | OUMs ... once | OUMs ... once |

# Week 12

***Week 12 is the same as WEEK 11***

## *'Getting there!'*

## Dr John Tickell's 91 Day Success Chart

*At the completion of each week, transfer your weekly Livinglife points to the Scoreboard on the inside back cover*

| ACE | Week 13 | M | T | W | T | F | S | S | My Total | Goal | Max |
|---|---|---|---|---|---|---|---|---|---|---|---|
| | | | | | | | | | | **Living*life* Points** | |
| A1 | Did I do my walk today? 2 points per day – Goal: 14 points per week. *If you walk minimum of 5 days per week – score 4 bonus points* | | | | | | | | | 14 | 14 |
| A2 | Did I do my strength work today? 1 point per day – Goal: 4 or 5 points per week | | | | | | | | | 5 | 7 |
| A3 | Did I do my OUMs today? 1 point per day – Goal: 4 or 5 points per week | | | | | | | | | 5 | 7 |
| | **ACTIVITY TOTALS** | | | | | | | | | **24** | **28** |
| E1 | Did I eat/nibble my 15 Plant Foods today? 2 points per day – Goal: 12 points per week | | | | | | | | | 12 | 14 |
| E2 | Did I do the 2/3, 1/3 routine today? 1 point per day – Goal: 6 points per week | | | | | | | | | 6 | 7 |
| E3 | Did I eat breakfast today? 1 point per day – Goal: 6 points per week | | | | | | | | | 6 | 7 |
| | **EATING TOTALS** | | | | | | | | | **24** | **28** |
| C1 | Did I have a laugh and give someone a hug today? 1 point per day – Goal: 6 points per week | | | | | | | | | 6 | 7 |
| C2 | Did I do some deep breathing and another relaxation thing today? 1 point per day – Goal: 6 points per week | | | | | | | | | 6 | 7 |
| C3 | Did I have a good sleep last night? 1 point per day – Goal: 6 points per week | | | | | | | | | 6 | 7 |
| C4 | Did I do something good for, or be nice to someone else today? 1 point per day – Goal: 6 points per week | | | | | | | | | 6 | 7 |
| | **COPING TOTALS** | | | | | | | | | **24** | **28** |
| | **WEEKLY GRAND TOTAL** | | | | | | | | | **72** | **84** |

*Switch-On weeks – aim at minimum of 60 LLPs per week*

*Switch-Off weeks – why not aim at the same number of LLPs?*

# Week 13 - Activity Schedule

Please mark these sessions in your diary - now - for this coming week.
Make the appointments with yourself.
The B.A.T and OUMs are laid out for you on Pages 143 and 150.

| | **Monday Day 1** | **Tuesday Day 2** | **Wednesday Day 3** | **Thursday Day 4** | **Friday Day 5** | **Saturday Day 6** | **Sunday Day 7** |
|---|---|---|---|---|---|---|---|
| 1.5% | | Walk<br>30 min. | Walk<br>30 min. | Walk<br>30 min. | | Walk<br>30 min. | Walk<br>30 min |
| SBW | | BAT<br>Exercises<br>Sets: 2<br>Reps: 10 | BAT<br>Exercises<br>Sets: 2<br>Reps: 10 | BAT<br>Exercises<br>Sets: 2<br>Reps: 10 | | BAT<br>Exercises<br>Sets: 2<br>Reps: 10 | BAT<br>Excercises<br>Sets: 2<br>Reps: 10 |
| OUMs | | OUMs<br>... once | OUMs<br>... once | OUMs<br>... once | | OUMs<br>... once | OUMs<br>... once |

# Week 13

***You're on the home stretch and you're eating REAL food.***

# Recipes

### *Breakfast Museli*

Buy a muesli base containing these ingredients - wheat flakes, oats and barley. Add chopped Brazil nuts, sultanas (or raisins) and sunflower seeds - all organic of course and store the mixture in an airtight container. Put ¾ of a cup of the muesli mixture into a bowl and add chopped apple, chopped dried apricot or any fresh fruit that's in season. Pour over half a cup of low fat milk or two tablespoons of low fat yoghurt. (If you are milk intolerant, use apple juice or orange juice instead).

### *Apricot and Cinnamon Porridge*

- ½ cup of instant porridge (traditional rolled oats)
- ¾ cup of skim milk (skinny milk) or low fat soy milk
- 4 dried or fresh apricots, chopped
- 2 teaspoons golden syrup
- a pinch of ground cinnamon

Simmer porridge and milk together for 4-5 minutes and stir out any lumps as it thickens - a little water may be added to get your required texture. Stir in golden syrup and cinnamon - serve in a bowl and sprinkle with chopped apricots.

### *No Yolk Omelette*

- 90 grams (3 ½ ounces) asparagus, trimmed or asparagus tips
- 90 grams (3 ½ ounces) of chopped fresh spinach
- Salt and ground black pepper
- 4 egg whites
- ½ teaspoon of sunflower oil

Steam or microwave the asparagus and the spinach and drain - season with pepper and salt.

Whisk egg whites until frothy and pouring consistency.

Heat oil in small non-stick pan, swirling it around until it covers the bottom in a thin film. Pour in omelette mixture and cook over low/ medium heat for 2-3 minutes until the bottom is firm. Slide omelette top side down on the asparagus and spinach and cook for another 2/3 minutes until the bottom is set and the asparagus and spinach is golden brown.

### ***Pancakes Supreme***

- 1¼ cups ground oatmeal
- 1¼ cups whole wheat pastry flour
- 1 tablespoon baking powder
- 2 tablespoons sugar
- 1 tablespoon vegetable oil
- ¾ cup blueberries
- 2½ cups water

Lightly mix all the ingredients in large bowl and leave 5 to 10 minutes to rise. It's important to mix the batter just enough to moisten, as over mixing will make the pancakes tough. Gently fold down. Leave again for 5 to 10 minutes if you have the time and gently fold down again. This second fold down and wait step is not crucial. Cook at medium to medium high heat on an oiled skillet or fry pan until golden, carefully breaking any large lumps with spatula. Serve immediately.

### ***Deluxe Tuna Sandwich***

Tuna sandwich with multi grain bread (for home or packed lunches)

*Tuna spread:*

- Mix to a paste 200 grams (7 ounces) canned tuna - drained
- 1½ tablespoons of low fat mayonnaise
- 2 tablespoons of finely chopped celery
- dash of Worcestershire sauce
- 2 teaspoons of chilli sauce
- 1 tablespoon fresh lemon juice

Mix will be sufficient for four sandwiches.

Spread mix on multi grain bread and top with thin slices of tomato, beetroot and cucumber.

***Minestrone Soup***

- 1 large clove garlic
- 2 medium potatoes
- 2 large carrots
- 2 pumpkin wedges
- 2 zucchini
- 1 stick celery
- 1 parsnip
- 1 brown onion
- 1 large leek
- 5-6 cups beef stock
- 2 large diced tomatoes
- 2 bay leaves
- 1 tablespoon canola spread
- black pepper
- 1 can red kidney beans (strained)
- 250 grams frozen baby peas

Melt canola in large pot. When hot, add crushed garlic and sliced potatoes, carrots, pumpkin, zucchini, celery, parsnip, onion and leek. Any other vegetable of your choice may be added.

Stir for about 3 minutes. Add diced tomatoes, beef stock, bay leaves and black pepper. Bring to the boil and then gently simmer until vegetables are just cooked. Add kidney beans and peas. Bring to the boil again and then remove from heat.

Discard bay leaves.

Optional – sprinkle small amount of grated low fat cheese on each bowl of soup.

***Japanese Miso Soup***

- 5 cups of water
- 3-4 tablespoons of Aka Miso (red soy bean paste)
  (Miso comes in a variety of flavours, textures and colours. Generally white types are sweet, red types are salty - usually found in refrigerated section of deli or supermarket).
- 1 packet or 3 tablespoons - dried shaved Bonito flakes (Bonito flakes are thin small flakes shaved from Bonito tuna that has been smoked, dried, and fermented).
- 1 teaspoon of instant dashi (Bonito soup stock)
- 3 scallions chopped
- 500 grams (1 lb) of cubed lean pork meat, or chicken if you wish
- 6 to 8 dried Shiitake mushrooms
- ½ cake of tofu cut into small squares
- 1-2 bundles of somen (a very thin white noodle)

Add pork or chicken to water in saucepan and cook until tender. Remove excess oil with a separator. Add additional water if necessary to make about 5 cups. Meanwhile soak dried Shiitake mushrooms in warm water until tender, then rinse - cut out and discard stems and slice thinly. Add to pork broth, bring to boil and add miso, Bonito flakes, dashi, scallions and tofu. Reduce heat and simmer 5 minutes. Cook somen to package directions (2-3 minutes). Pour soup mixture over somen, top with fresh cut scallions and serve.

***Poached Atlantic Salmon***

- 1 fillet of Atlantic salmon - approx. 200 grams (7 ounces)
- 2 cups of orange juice
- 1 chicken stock cube
- 2 small white potatoes
- 2 heads of broccoli
- Generous serve of spinach (fresh or frozen)
- Green peas

Boil or microwave the potatoes and steam or microwave the vegetables. Pour the orange juice into a fry pan over moderate heat, add chicken stock cube and blend. Add salmon fillet and poach until the orange flesh (which is immersed in the orange juice) loses its colour, turn the fillet over and continue poaching until whole fillet has lost its colour. This will take no more than 12 minutes. Serve fish, pour over orange juice and add vegetables.

***Baked Fish with Lemon Tahini (sesame seed paste)***

- 1 fillet of white fish - Ocean Perch, Orange Roughie, Coral Trout or similar
- Sea salt and black pepper
- 1 teaspoon olive oil
- 1 dessertspoon of Tahini paste
- 1 tablespoon of lemon juice
- Grated zest of ½ lemon
- 1 tablespoon of low fat yoghurt
- ¼ clove of garlic
- 1 tablespoon of fresh chopped parsley

Sprinkle fillet on both sides with a little salt and leave to stand for about 30 minutes.

Grill the fish for 6-7 minutes each side whilst whisking the sauce ingredients (except for the parsley) with a tablespoon of water to make a smooth paste. Add the parsley and mix well.

Heat oven to 230 degrees.

Place fish in ovenproof dish, spoon over sauce and bake for 10 minutes or until the sauce bubbles and starts to brown.

Garnish with thin slices of lemon and fresh parsley.

Serve with boiled white potato and steamed broccoli, cauliflower, Brussels sprouts, peas and green beans.

### ***Chicken and Apricot Sauce***

Served with potato, steamed beans, broccoli, carrots, Brussels sprouts

- 200 gram (7 ounces) skinless breast of chicken.

Cook in non stick fry pan with 1 tablespoon extra virgin olive oil over medium to high heat, turning chicken as it cooks until all sides are golden brown. Test by slicing with knife to ensure flesh is all white with no streaks of red.

*Apricot sauce:*

- 500 grams (18 ounces) canned apricots in syrup
- ¼ cup brown sugar
- 1 tablespoon cornstarch
- 1 tablespoon lemon juice
- 1 tablespoon brown mustard
- 1 teaspoon Worcestershire sauce
- 1 clove garlic
- ½ cup chopped dried apricots
- 1 tablespoon butter

In blender or food processor combine apricots in syrup, brown sugar, cornstarch, lemon juice, brown mustard, Worcestershire sauce, and garlic clove. Process until smooth. Pour mixture into a saucepan and stir in chopped dried apricots.

Cook, stirring until thickened, about 2 minutes. Remove from heat and stir in butter. Plate the cooked chicken, pour over enough sauce to cover, add potato and steamed vegetables and serve. Refrigerate the surplus sauce for later use.

### ***Vegetable Casserole***

- 300 grams (10 ounces) green beans
- 2 medium potatoes
- 1 dessertspoon cream (or low fat milk)
- 1 slice low fat cheese (1 single)
- 120 grams (4 ounces) button mushrooms
- 1 red pepper
- 2 rashers rindless bacon (optional) - remove all fat

***Sauce***

1 can crushed tomatoes
olive oil
1 clove garlic
2 tablespoons water
a pinch of sea salt, add pepper
1 teaspoon Worcestershire sauce
1 tablespoon chopped parsley

Peel potatoes and slice thinly. Place in shallow dish and sprinkle cream (or low fat milk) over top. Cook covered in microwave for 5 minutes. Remove and sprinkle with the cheese (broken into small pieces).

Top, tail and string beans - cut into pieces. Cook covered in microwave for 3 minutes.

Slice mushrooms and pepper thinly and combine with the cooked beans. Spread vegetable mixture over potatoes.

Heat pan, add just enough olive oil to coat base of pan. Cook crushed garlic and sliced onion until soft. Add salt, pepper, parsley, Worcestershire sauce, water and entire contents of crushed tomatoes can. Heat through. Pour sauce over vegetables. Cook, uncovered in microwave for 8 minutes. Add diced, cooked bacon, if desired.

***Char-grilled Kangaroo Fillet***

Served with wok scorched vegetables and Vietnamese mint (Serves 4)

**A** 4 x 170g kangaroo fillets
- 4 tablespoons soy sauce (from an Asian Supermarket)
- 3 cloves garlic – peeled, smashed and chopped
- 1 fresh red chilli – split, seeded, chopped
- 2 tablespoon finely sliced young lemon grass

**B** 2 good size head broccoli (cut into florets)
- 150g snow peas cut on the slant
- 1 red capsicum seeded and sliced
- 2 baby bok choy – roughly chopped
- 1 Spanish red onion sliced
- 50 ml extra virgin sesame oil
- 2 tablespoons chopped Vietnamese mint

1. Combine all ingredients in Section A together and allow to infuse.
2. Prepare all vegetables in Section B
3. Clean kangaroo fillet of any sinew if necessary. Rub with olive oil, season with salt and pepper. Char-grill on hot griddle for 3–4 minutes until medium rare. Remove and rest in a warm place.
4. Heat Sesame oil in wok, sear the vegetables, stirring over high hear for 2–3 minutes. Drizzle in sauce and toss to coat, check for taste, adjust if necessary, add Vietnamese mint.
Divide onto four warmed bowls top with sliced kangaroo fillet and serve.

*Recipe courtesy of Celebrity Chef, Phillip Mitchell from The Sebel Reef House, Palm Cove, North Queensland.*

# Where to now? - Beyond 91 days

After 91 DAYS, if you have been true to yourself, then we are sailing into smoother waters.

What have we achieved?

> I trust that **Activity** has become part of your life and that the human machine (you) is grateful for its walking, its stretching and its well-toned muscles.

> I trust that you appreciate that **good food** is good – it heals, it provides energy and that if you want to eat food that other humans have wrecked – then do it just now and then and have only small amounts.

> I trust that you are **Coping** a little better – the relaxation things, the 'f's back in your life, and a good self-image. That's **you** liking **you**.

It doesn't stop here. If you've done well – set some new goals. If you've fallen a little short, then set some new goals. Achievement is the cornerstone of living.

Step by step.

And remember the **Four Aces**. If you hold the Four Aces in your pack of cards, you can be truly happy.

After all what's the ultimate aim in life?

**Happiness.**

# SEALED SECTION

The Great Australian Diet:
The Atkins Alternative
Dr John Tickell

>

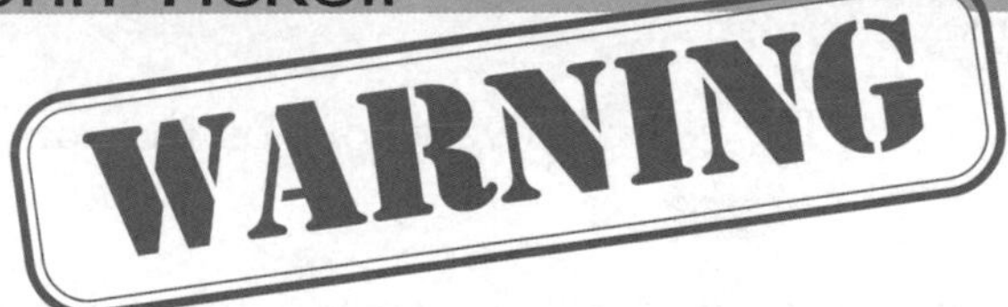


This section may contain material
that makes a lot of sense.

# What other diet books don't tell you

So why do we really put on weight?

Well, there is so much crappy stuff happening in our lives today.

That's the real reason.

It's not just the bad food.

All these different pressures on us to do this and do that.

Pressures on the kids to make decisions (and they probably won't discuss most of their problems with you).

Pressure on our relationships, because every magazine tells us what should be happening, where we're going wrong, what we need to be doing to be 'perfect'.

Too much information.

Then there's 'The News' – every hour, on the hour. All bad news.

What we need to do is get rid of a lot of this stuff – at least three-quarters of it.

Put your worries in the little boxes on the side of your brain and just let them out now and then.

Don't let it get to you.

Forget 'The News' for a week or so.

The other thing that's happening out there is change.

Everything is going too fast.

Only about 10% of people are excited by change and 90% of us are threatened by change because it is so unpredictable.

Anyway, people with **routine** in their lives – live the longest.

What we need to do is have some fun. You've just got to have a laugh now and then.

My wife tells me this …

*'Go down to the pub and have a drink with the boys.'*

I say to my wife ...

*'Thanks, and you go out to dinner with the girls and have a good bitch and a good laugh.'*

The kids are a worry.

Where are they?

What are they doing?

What time is it?

They should be home by now.

And the girls are getting their periods so young these days.

Why?

Same reasons – more fat, more hormones, less vegetables, less exercise.

Does it matter?

Well a century ago, they started at 17 or 18 and now it can be as young as 12 or 13!

That's six years times 12 cycles ... equals 72 more shots of oestrogen into the system ... and that means a higher risk of breast cancer.

Scary, huh?

Do you like drinking Coke?

The other diet book authors would be horrified if they read this.

Your brain is fed by glucose. Glucose is sugar in the blood stream.

Carbohydrates actually break down in the body to mainly glucose.

Glucose make the brain feel good. It makes it fire up and helps your brain think smarter.

So do I drink Coke?

Don't tell anyone this, but yes, every now and then when I'm really thirsty or if I need a kick start. But I never drink the whole can – just two or three mouthfuls and then I tip the rest on the garden or the roadway.

It costs the same whether you drink the whole can or a third of the can.

This all comes down to being in control.

I was extremely fortunate to be able to write a book with a hero of mine – the legendary Jack Nicklaus – the greatest golfer the game has ever seen.

He told me that when he flies in a helicopter he insists on a second set of controls, just in case something goes wrong with the pilot.

Nicklaus can't fly a chopper too well but at least he can get it down on the ground.

He wants to be in control.

Which brings me to another point.

It's a great idea to have heros in our lives. Kids with posters of their heros stuck on their bedroom wall are inspired, every morning they wake up. It's great!

As adults, the pictures on our walls are landscapes and other things. Maybe we should do the hero routine so **we** are inspired each morning – inspired to go out and do some good for the world.

Mid mornings, I like to get out of the office and go down the local café for a break. I'll order a cappuccino.

When I'm in a creative mode and writing and thinking about stuff, I can't do it closed in by four walls in the office. I need to get out.

I ask them to do the cappuccino or latte with low fat milk and if they say 'too hard' then I go for half non-fat (skim) and half regular. Most times they'll do that.

If you want a sugar hit, sprinkle ¾ teaspoon of sugar on the fluff. Don't worry about it – ¾ teaspoon of sugar is only 13 calories, so once a day is not going to kill you.

Money is a huge cause of stress – usually not enough of it, but some rich guys can get stressed with too much of it (we wish). And when we are stressed, that's a trigger to eat.

Boredom is another trigger. If you're bored, go for a bike ride. Haven't got a bike? – well get one.

If you haven't got enough money for a short break or holiday then stop buying so much junk (or beer or smokes) and put $10 in a jar every day for three months. That's plenty to buy an el-cheapo airfare and a few days by a beach.

Or get a part-time job for two or three months.

Have a green tea every morning – buy the little tea-bags with green tea and jasmine.

You don't need milk or sugar. After a while it tastes sensational by itself.

If you eat a cooked breakfast day after day after day (because some diet book told you to do that) – you feel like GLUG.

Sometimes I indulge when I'm away, but your body sort of just doesn't feel right if you keep doing it.

It's supposed to make you lose weight but honestly, the people I visit in the East just don't do that.

It doesn't make sense.

And if you actually could see what happens in those tiny little coronary arteries (the ones that keep your heart alive) after a big fatty meal, you wouldn't go there too often.

A bit like smoking. If your lungs were hanging on the outside of your body and you could see all the shit accumulating, you would never have another cigarette in you life.

There are lots of tricks – like just have a quarter of the yolk when you eat an egg.

That's all you need for 100% taste.

What makes you feel good – apart from food?

Movies.

Feel good movies or chase 'em, shoot 'em, kill 'em dead movies?

Whichever answer (a) or (b) tells me a lot about you.

There's plenty of (b) in the news every day so why do you need to watch it night after night on TV?

And those computer games where guys kill each other and blow things to bits and you win by eliminating lots of people ... it doesn't affect the kids, the experts say.

Don't believe them. They're dead wrong.

So what's the bottom line?

If you lived in a village, worked in the fields, did some fishing most days, ate kangaroo meat and vegetables, had a glass of wine and hugged the kids – you wouldn't be fat or even overweight.

It really comes down to how close you can get to what I've said.

And you need some fun and excitement in your life as well.

**Lighten up folks**.

It's the crap in our lives that make us fat.

The fries, the goodies, the synthetic snacks, the negative stress, the frustration, the sitting on our butt stuff.

- Eat some REAL food will you? Low H.I. and MOVE!
- Walk, walk, walk
- Climb stairs – convince yourself and your thighs that you **love** stairs

> Dance
> ... give your 600 muscles something to do every waking hour
> SBWs and OUMs – do them
> Take two deep breaths every hour
> Laugh
> Love your kids
> Love your parents
> Celebrate life every day

Thank you

Dr John Tickell

**The Great Australian Diet is the best alternative for REAL LIFE**

## To contact Dr John Tickell

For speaking engagements and corporate presentations

*Email: drjohntickell@drjohntickell.com*

To order books, DVDs, videos, newsletters and for general information on health, stress and nutrition, go to

*www.drjohntickell.com*

A brilliant idea ...

Subscribe to Dr John Tickell's monthly newsletter 'Livinglife'. For your free copy, go to

*www.drjohntickell.com*